Multiple Choice Questions for the MRCP

Pankaj Joshi

MB, ChB (Natal), MRCP (UK), FICA (USA)

Part-time Consultant Physician – Kalafong and Laudium Hospitals,
Pretoria;
Fellow of the Royal Society of Medicine, London.
Formerly Consultant Physician, Departments of Medicine,
Baragwanath and Johannesburg General Hospitals and the University
of Witwatersrand, Johannesburg, South Africa

BUTTERWORTHS
London - Boston - Durban - Singapore - Sydney - Toronto - Wellington

First published 1982
Reprinted 1985

© **Butterworth & Co (Publishers) Ltd 1982**

British Library Cataloguing in Publication Data

Joshi, Pankaj
    Multiple choice questions for the MRCP.
    1. Pathology—Problems, exercises, etc.
    I. Title
    616'.0076   RB119

ISBN 0–407–00247–2

Library of Congress Cataloging in Publication Data

Joshi, Pankaj.
    Multiple choice questions for the MRCP.

    Bibliography: p.
    Includes index.
    1. Internal medicine–Examinations, questions, etc.   I. Title.
    [DHLM: 1. Medicine–examination questions. W. 18 J83m]
    RC5B.J67 1985   616'.0076   85–11683
    ISBN 0–407–00247–2

Typeset by Phoenix Photosetting
Printed in England by
Camelot Press Ltd, Southampton

Multiple Choice Questions for the MRCP

To the memory of my brother
Gajanan
who was and will always remain
a tower of constant inspiration to me

Foreword

This admirable collection of multiple choice questions and answers is mainly intended for candidates preparing themselves for higher examinations in medicine. The questions should be answered in writing—without peeping—and corrected later by referring to the answers given. Attempting self-audit in this way is a valuable exercise in medical education. It should prove a rewarding form of study provided the central role of bedside medicine is not neglected. The questions have been carefully selected by the author and checked from standard texts and by discussion with many colleagues who are practising clinicians and teachers of medicine.

The author, Pankaj Joshi, was once my student and was a consultant physician on my firm at the General Hospital, Johannesburg. His knowledge and diligence are reflected in these pages. I wish him and his book the success so well deserved.

E. B. Adams, MD, FRCP
Emeritus Professor of Medicine,
University of Natal; Principal Physician,
General Hospital, Johannesburg

v

Preface

The multiple choice question is a relatively new innovation in the examination format. It thus requires a fresh approach, a new orientation and a different technique from the conventional essay type—Question and Answer—examination. There are, indeed, many pitfalls which may trap the unwary, and this book draws the candidates attention to these.

While this book is intended for candidates taking any multiple choice form of examination in the discipline of internal medicine, it is directed primarily to the candidate sitting for Part 1 of the MRCP (UK) examination.

This book is no substitute for a sound knowledge of medicine, which is clearly the *sine qua non* for any examination. No pretension is, therefore, made to provide all the facts which are necessary to pass the examination. All the questions appearing in this monograph are supported by cross-reference to a bibliographical reference list which is included. A special, relatively large section, is included at the end which correlates common topics and relates observations such as causes of papilloedema and causes of Raynaud's phenomenon.

This monograph is thus set out as a guided approach to the preparation for the examination, an approach to the specific techniques, and to the topics and questions requiring particular attention. It is fervently hoped that such an approach will smooth the path for the aspirant candidate.

Pankaj Joshi

Acknowledgements

It is a great pleasure to express my thanks to: Professor Leo Schamroth, MD, DSc., FRCP (Ed), FRCPG, FACC, FRS (SA), Chief Physician, Baragwanath Hospital, Johannesburg, for guiding me in the preparation of this book, for his constant constructive criticism and for his never-ending encouragement; Professor Asher Dubb, MB, ChB, Dip. Med (SA), Principal Physician, Baragwanath Hospital, for reviewing the entire manuscript, correcting spelling and grammatical errors, pointing out ambiguously phrased questions and making invaluable suggestions; Drs D.M. Mzamane, MB, ChB, FCP (SA), S. Hurwitz, MB, ChB, FCP (SA), D. Saffer, MB, ChB, MRCP (London), P.L.A. Bill, MB, ChB, FCP (SA), MRCP (UK), for thoroughly reviewing and correcting sections of the manuscript, and Dr R.H.C. Ming, MB, ChB, for attempting all the questions and rechecking the answers with me, all my colleagues who provided me constantly with encouragement and support; my wife, Nazeeha, and my children who very patiently and understandingly prompted me along in the completion of this book.

Acknowledgements are due also to Reedprint Ltd., Windsor, UK, for permission to reproduce the specimen answer sheets.

Pankaj Joshi

Contents

Chapter 1
The MRCP Multiple Choice Examination

The structure of the MRCP multiple choice examination

The MRCP (UK) examination has to be taken in two parts. Part I of the examination is dealt with in this book. Part II of the examination has a written section and a clinical section. The written section includes a section that requires answers to 20 projected slides of physical signs, dermatological conditions, radiographs, histological and haematological photographs, a section on 10 data for interpretation, and finally a section on 4 'grey' cases, that is case histories (usually including one paediatric case history) with questions relating to differential diagnoses, management and therapeutic approaches. These are all compulsory. Further, an oral examination lasting 20 minutes has to be attended. This is followed by a clinical examination, in which one long case has to be examined over one hour, followed by its presentation and discussion, and then a series of short cases are shown over 20 minutes. The written section is separated from the oral and clinical sections by a period of about 4 to 6 weeks.

Part I of the examination is held three times a year. For further details see Appendix.

The Part I Examination

A maximum of four attempts are allowed for this part of the examination. The examination is written over 2½ hours and

1

comprises one paper of 60 multiple choice questions. The questions are in book form with the answer sheets folded at the end of the book. Each initial statement (or stem) is followed by five possible completions (or items) listed as A,B,C,D, and E. These have to be answered as True, False or Do Not Know. One mark (+1) is awarded for each correct answer. A correct answer is a true statement indicated as true in the answer, or a false statement indicated as false in the answer. One mark is deducted (−1) for each incorrect answer, that is, a true statement indicated as false and vice versa. A zero mark is awarded for each Do Not Know answer. The time allotted is adequate and there should be no urgency to complete the paper.

The answer sheets contain a row of boxes for each question, the odd-numbered questions are on the left and the even-numbered on the right. Specimen sheets are presented at the end of each examination in Chapter 2. Each box refers to a single item and is numbered accordingly (i.e. 1A, 1B, 1C, etc.). In each box there are 3 rectangles labelled T (True), F (False) and D (Do Not Know). You should indicate whether you think a particular item is true or false by filling in the appropriate rectangle; if you are uncertain you must fill in the rectangles labelled D because the computer checks its efficiency by ensuring it has sensed a pencil indication for every response. Thus, you must fill in one of the rectangles in each of the 300 boxes. Failure to do so results in rejection of your answer sheet by the computer.

The techniques for the multiple choice examination

1. It is essential to read the questions carefully and thoroughly to avoid misinterpretation of what is being asked. This cannot be overemphasized.
2. You must be absolutely certain you are not marking the wrong boxes—this would be most unfortunate. Allow for enough time to recheck your entries.
3. Do not look for trick questions in the examination, as this is not intended by the examiners.
4. You may erase an answer by using the eraser provided, and then fill in another rectangle. To avoid too many erasures on the answer sheet, you are advised to indicate your choices of true and false items in the question book itself in the first

instance, before transferring them to the answer sheets.

Use this technique when answering the questions in this monograph so that you may become familiar with the format and thereby gain adequate practice in allowing sufficient time to make the final entries.

5. It is important to remember that there is no restriction on the number of true or false items in a question. It is possible for all the items in a question to be true, or all to be false. Thus, each item of a question should be answered on its own merit independently, disregarding the preceding or succeeding items (or completions) of the questions.

6. Nobody is, unfortunately, certain what the pass mark for the examination is. Therefore, the following approach is suggested. The candidate is advised first to answer ONLY those questions about which he is certain of the answers. Any answers about which he is uncertain should be left unanswered until later. The total number of answered questions should be calculated. If the total is above 210, there should be no real problem in passing the examination. There must be very few examinations, if any, in which a mark of 70% would fail a candidate! If the total is about 200, there is, I believe, still a reasonable safety margin for passing the examination, and the unanswered questions should be reviewed. The candidate now will often be able to recall or even work out some of the answers.

If the total count is much less, the candidate should answer only those questions about which he feels reasonably certain, where the guess is a calculated one, and not one where just a 50 : 50 chance is taken. Blind guessing is NOT advisable, as marks already earned will be lost if the answers are wrong.

7. Any question that includes the word NEVER or ALWAYS should be answered in the affirmative only if you are absolutely sure of the answer. Many of the answers to these questions frequently turn out to be false!

8. There are some terms used in the multiple choice examination that are commonly confused or misinterpreted. These are defined here for clarification:

(a) The terms PATHOGNOMONIC and SPECIFIC indicate features that occur in the condition named, and in no other condition.

(b) A RECOGNIZED FEATURE is a feature that has been well documented as occurring in the condition under discussion.

(c) A CHARACTERISTIC feature is one that occurs frequently and lends strong support to the diagnosis.

(d) TYPICAL is a word similar in meaning to characteristic and is used interchangeably.

(e) The term MAJORITY is taken to mean greater than 50%.

Ten typical model examinations are presented in this book. The distribution of the different sections in the individual papers has been guided by:

(a) the guidelines presented in the Royal College of Physicians Symposium titled MRCP 1977 appearing in the *British Medical Journal*, **1**, 217–220;

(b) the recent decision taken by the Royal College of Physicians to increase gradually the total number of basic science questions in the examinations. In a personal communication with the Royal College of Physicians of London (3rd June, 1981), I have been informed that the proportion of basic science questions will increase gradually over the next 2 to 3 years until the proportion reaches about 30%. However, the basic science questions will be of exactly the same type as those being set presently.

The above format is being adhered to to simulate the actual examination as closely as possible in its presently intended form.

At the end of each examination paper an answer sheet is provided, similar to the ones in the actual examination. This has been included to give the candidate not only an opportunity for self-assessment, but also to get practice at what will be expected in Part I of the examination.

To derive maximum benefit from this book, the reader is advised to tackle the model examinations under simulated examination conditions, allowing a maximum time of 2½ hours. A mark for every correct entry should then be scored, a mark for incorrect entries subtracted and a zero score awarded for any Do Not Know entries made.

Chapter 2
Model Examination Papers; Each with Following Referenced Answers

Examination 1
(Time allotted: 2½ hours)

1. **The following statements are true regarding hyperuricaemia:**
   A It may be caused by the treatment of hypertension
   B There is a higher association with hyperlipoproteinaemia than can be explained by chance
   C In 25% of gouty patients urinary uric acid values are excessive
   D It is rarely idiopathic
   E Treatment with allopurinol is contraindicated if renal failure is present

2. **In the diagnosis of pulmonary aspergilloma:**
   A Serum precipitins to aspergillosis are strongly positive
   B Sputum cultures are characteristically positive
   C Skin sensitivity tests are usually negative
   D The chest x-ray shows a ball shadow in a cavity which shifts with a change in position of the patient
   E Pronounced blood eosinophilia is usually found

3. **In systemic sclerosis:**
   A Oesophageal strictures are seen in the majority of patients
   B Pneumothorax is a recognized complication
   C Some patients may rapidly develop malignant hypertension
   D Cold agglutinins are seen in 25% of patients
   E There is a threefold increase in prevalence in coal miners

4. **Psoriasis may be aggravated by:**
   A Antimalarial drugs
   B Antimitotic drugs
   C Sulphonamides
   D Pregnancy
   E Salicylates

5. **Eosinophilia occurs with:**
   A Polyarteritis nodosa
   B Adrenal cortical hyperfunction
   C Wegener's granulomatosis
   D *Toxocara canis* infection
   E Scarlet fever

6. **Renal calcification is a recognized feature of:**
   A Medullary sponge kidneys
   B Renal tuberculosis
   C Sarcoidosis
   D Sickle-cell anaemia
   E Secondary hyperparathyroidism

7. **Varicella is associated with:**
   A A very itchy rash
   B An incubation period of 14–21 days
   C A rash which first appears on the trunk
   D A rash in the mouth
   E A rash which occurs in crops

8. **Proteinuria in rheumatoid arthritis may be caused by:**
   A Analgesic nephropathy
   B Renal involvement by the disease *per se*
   C Amyloidosis
   D Myocrisin therapy
   E Therapy with non–steroidal anti–inflammatory agents

9. **Recognized side–effects of phenytoin therapy include:**
   A Haemolytic anaemia
   B Macrocytic anaemia due to vitamin B_{12} deficiency
   C Gum hypertrophy
   D Generalized lymphadenopathy
   E Hypocalcaemia

10. **Phenylketonuria may be associated with:**
   A Diminished pigmentation of the hair, eyes and skin
   B An autosomal dominant inheritance
   C Higher incidence in boys
   D Heterozygous trait which is not injurious
   E Convulsions

11. **Reiter's disease is typically associated with:**
   A A positive anti–nuclear factor
   B Balanitis circinata
   C Conjunctivitis
   D Keratoderma blenorrhagica
   E Livedo reticularis

12. **In fibrocystic disease of the pancreas:**
   A Splenomegaly may be found
   B Frequent staphylococcal infections of the skin are seen
   C D-xylose absorption is impaired
   D The patient is in a positive nitrogen balance
   E There is an increased absorption of iron

13. **In Addison's disease the following values are low:**
    A   Serum sodium
    B   Urinary potassium
    C   Blood sugar
    D   Serum chloride
    E   Serum bicarbonate

14. **African Trypanosomiasis:**
    A   Is transmitted by both sexes of the tsetse fly
    B   Is unassociated with neurological symptoms in the first week
    C   Commonly produces posterior cervical lymphadenopathy
    D   May produce aplastic anaemia
    E   Responds favourably only to suramin therapy

15. **Cavitating lesions on the chest x-ray are typically seen with:**
    A   Staphylococcal pneumonia
    B   Klebsiella pneumonia
    C   Pulmonary embolism
    D   Pulmonary tuberculosis
    E   Sarcoidosis

16. **Lead poisoning in children commonly produces the following manifestations:**
    A   Severe anaemia
    B   Wrist drop
    C   Encephalopathy
    D   Papilloedema
    E   Basophilic stippling of red blood cells

17. **Side-effects of lithium carbonate therapy include:**
    A   Acquired ichthyosis
    B   Macrocytic anaemia
    C   Polyuria and polydipsia
    D   Deteriorating vision
    E   Tremors

18. **The following conditions are associated with intracerebral calcification:**
    A   Tuberous sclerosis
    B   Congenital toxoplasmosis
    C   Intracerebral secondaries
    D   Tuberculosis
    E   Inclusion body encephalitis

19. **Bilateral lower motor neurone seventh nerve lesions are seen in:**
    A   Guillain–Barré syndrome
    B   Sarcoidosis
    C   Leprosy
    D   Myasthenia gravis
    E   Pseudobulbar palsy

20. **Mid-diastolic murmurs over the mitral area may be heard in:**
    A   Left atrial myxoma
    B   Mitral stenosis with atrial fibrillation
    C   Aortic incompetence
    D   Acute rheumatic fever
    E   Organic pulmonary incompetence

21. **Tall R waves in V_1 on the electrocardiogram are produced by:**
    A   Right bundle branch block
    B   Ebstein's anomaly
    C   Wolff–Parkinson–White syndrome
    D   Acute pulmonary embolism
    E   True dextrocardia

22. **In motor neurone disease the following often occur:**
    A   Wasting of muscles
    B   Urinary incontinence
    C   Spastic paralysis
    D   Fasciculations
    E   Dementia

23. **The following conditions are associated with megaloblastic anaemia in patients with cancer:**
A   Treatment with alkylating agents
B   Post-irradiation
C   Secondary spread to the bone marrow
D   Hypersplenism
E   Coomb's positive haemolytic anaemia

24. **Inappropriate antidiuretic hormone production occurs with:**
A   Islet-cell carcinoma of the pancreas
B   Demethylchlortetracycline (Ledermycin) therapy
C   Meningitis
D   Camcolit (lithium carbonate) therapy
E   Oat-cell carcinoma of the bronchus

25. **Clinical features which favour primary hyperparathyroidism as opposed to the syndrome of non-metastatic hypercalcaemia of malignancy include:**
A   Polyuria and polydipsia
B   Nephrocalcinosis
C   Constipation
D   More acute onset
E   Presence of classic radiological bony features

26. **In cold-agglutinin haemolytic anaemia:**
A   The antibody is an IgM
B   Constitutional features with fevers and chills are common
C   Reticulocyte count is usually greater than 50%
D   Splenectomy is the treatment of choice
E   Raynaud's phenomenon results

27. **The following statements are true regarding the thyroid gland:**
    A The external branch of the superior laryngeal nerve is anterior to its upper pole
    B The superior thyroid artery arises from the external carotid artery
    C The whole gland may remain as a swelling at the tongue base
    D The gland is enclosed in the pretracheal fascia
    E The isthmus overlies the 5th and 6th tracheal rings

28. **Growth retardation is found in a child with:**
    A Severe maternal deprivation
    B Rickets
    C Hypothyroidism
    D Hurler's syndrome
    E Long-term penicillin therapy

29. **Physical signs simulating pneumonia may be produced by:**
    A Carcinoma of the bronchus
    B Acute pulmonary oedema
    C Moderate pleural effusion
    D Pulmonary infarction
    E Pulmonary fibrosis

30. **Congenital toxoplasmosis is characteristically associated with:**
    A Involvement of neonates in successive pregnancies
    B Bilateral chorioretinitis
    C Renal abnormalities
    D Calcification of the skull
    E Congenital cardiac lesions if fetus infected in the first trimester

31. **The following statements regarding chromosomes are true:**
    A   The normal number is 46
    B   Mosaicism is when an organism has cells with different numbers of chromosomes
    C   They are always identical in phenotypic cells
    D   If non-disjunction has occurred, then translocation must occur
    E   They may be used as markers in cancer

32. **Graves' disease (primary thyrotoxicosis) is characteristically:**
    A   Associated with exophthalmic ophthalmoplegia
    B   Associated with clubbing
    C   Found in young males
    D   Known to develop pretibial myxoedema following therapy
    E   Associated with fasciculations of the tongue

33. **Cataracts typically occur in:**
    A   Hypercalcaemia
    B   Ionizing radiation
    C   Toxoplasmosis
    D   Dystrophia myotonica
    E   Glaucoma

34. **The following statements suggest that the asthmatic attack is severe:**
    A   Pulsus paradoxus of 40 mmHg
    B   Peripheral cyanosis without central cyanosis
    C   Pulse rate of 98 per minute
    D   Inspiratory stridor
    E   Q–T prolongation on the electrocardiogram

35. **The following statements are true:**
  A   The geometric mean is always less than the arithmetic mean
  B   The Null hypothesis assumes that there is a significant difference between the population mean and the sample means, but that this should be ignored
  C   The square root of the variance is the standard deviation
  D   Sampling error is less in a stratified random sample than in a simple random sample
  E   The value of the variable which occurs with the greatest frequency is the median

36. **Aetiological factors of peptic ulcers include:**
  A   Smoking cigarettes
  B   Biliary cirrhosis
  C   Hypoparathyroidism
  D   Zollinger–Ellison syndrome
  E   Colchicine therapy

37. **Ducket Jones' major criteria for the diagnosis of rheumatic fever are:**
  A   Chorea gravidarum
  B   Tender nodules on the pretibial areas
  C   Arthritis of the proximal interphalangeal joints
  D   Erythema marginatum
  E   Osler's nodes

38. **Endogenous depression is characterized by:**
  A   Onset following loss of a loved one
  B   Difficulty in falling off to sleep
  C   Suicidal thoughts
  D   Rapid response to tricyclic antidepressant therapy
  E   Pathognomonic electroencephalographic (EEG) changes

39. **Extra-articular complications of rheumatoid arthritis include:**
   A Leucoerythroblastic anaemia
   B Pericardial effusion
   C Interstitial pulmonary fibrosis
   D Peripheral neuropathy
   E Cytoid bodies in the retina

40. **The types of liver disease in ulcerative colitis include:**
   A Primary biliary cirrhosis
   B Portal pyaemia
   C Chronic active hepatitis
   D Fatty infiltration
   E Acute fulminant hepatitis

41. **The following drugs are bacteriostatic in normal doses:**
   A Tetracyclines
   B Cephalosporins
   C Co-trimoxazole
   D Erythromycin
   E Amoxicillin

42. **Patients with ankylosing spondylitis:**
   A Are exclusively young males
   B May be prevented from developing calcification of the vertebral ligaments by early steroid therapy
   C May have associated peripheral joint involvement
   D Die more frequently of leukaemia
   E Have radiological sacroiliitis as an early sign

43. **The following factors predispose to urinary tract infections:**
   A Urinary obstruction
   B Diabetes mellitus
   C Hyperkalaemia
   D Long-term tetracycline therapy
   E Pregnancy

44. **A 45-year-old male presents with a history of vertigo and faintness associated with sweating. The differential diagnosis must include:**
   A   Hyperventilation
   B   Hyperglycaemia
   C   Zollinger–Ellison syndrome
   D   Phaeochromocytoma
   E   Paroxysmal tachycardia

45. **Recognized toxic side-effects of colchicine include:**
   A   Convulsions
   B   Severe abdominal pains
   C   Haemorrhagic gastroenteritis
   D   Ascending paralysis of the central nervous system
   E   Photosensitivity reactions

46. **The rash in:**
   A   Measles appears on the 2nd day
   B   Varicella appears on the 1st day
   C   Smallpox appears on the 3rd day
   D   Secondary syphilis is usually vesicular
   E   Erythema marginatum is itchy

47. **Recurrent sterile meningitis is recognized with:**
   A   Behçet's disease
   B   Guillain–Barré syndrome
   C   Sarcoidosis
   D   Vogt–Koyanagi–Harada disease
   E   Lepromatous leprosy

48. **Sudden loss of vision occurs in:**
   A   Bilateral anterior cerebral artery thromboses
   B   High dose chloroquine therapy
   C   Temporal arteritis
   D   Massive gastrointestinal haemorrhage
   E   Retinal detachment

49. **Recognized causes of haematemesis are:**
   A   Salicylate ingestion
   B   Oral iron tablets overdosage
   C   Severe burns
   D   Ménétrièr's disease
   E   Nasogastric suction

50. **Congestive cardiomyopathy typically presents with:**
   A   An ejection systolic murmur best heard at the lower left parasternal border
   B   Biventricular enlargement
   C   Jerky pulse
   D   Systemic embolic phenomena
   E   Sudden death

51. **Narcolepsy:**
   A   Should be treated with chlorpromazine
   B   Is associated with cataplexy
   C   Is due to infection with Trypanosomes
   D   Is associated with hypnagogic hallucinations
   E   Patients may have associated sleep paralysis

52. **The following drugs cause fluid retention:**
   A   Salicylates in high doses
   B   Chlorpromazine
   C   Phenobarbitone
   D   Phenylbutazone
   E   Carbenoxolone sodium

53. **Primary generalized epilepsy is characterized by:**
   A   Onset with an olfactory aura
   B   Seeing halos around lights preceding the onset of the seizures
   C   Development of postictal hemiplegia
   D   A three-cycle-per-second wave and spike form on EEG
   E   A positive family history

54. **Generalized lymphadenopathy is described in:**
   A   Chronic phenylbutazone therapy
   B   Sarcoidosis
   C   Hepatic cirrhosis
   D   Infectious mononucleosis
   E   Lymphadenoma

55. **Asbestosis is associated with the following:**
   A   Development of clubbing
   B   Upper and midzonal pulmonary fibrosis
   C   Increased incidence of bronchogenic carcinoma
   D   Increased incidence of peritoneal mesothelioma
   E   Hepatic fibrosis

56. **Hepatic failure may produce:**
   A   Positive alpha fetoprotein in the serum
   B   A characteristic tremor
   C   High output cardiac failure
   D   Hypoglycaemia
   E   Central cyanosis

57. **The following factors affect the glomerular filtration rate:**
   A   Hypoproteinaemia
   B   Presence of cystitis
   C   Changes in renal blood flow
   D   Alterations in the transport maximum
   E   Changes in hydrostatic pressure in Bowman's capsule

58. **Psychiatric presentation may be found in:**
   A   Myxoedema
   B   Acute intermittent porphyria
   C   Motor neurone disease
   D   Thyrotoxicosis
   E   Syringomyelia

59. **Causes of carpal tunnel syndrome include:**
     A   Ochronosis
     B   Acromegaly
     C   Type IIa familial hypercholesterolaemia
     D   Rheumatoid arthritis
     E   Pregnancy

60. **Polyclonal gammopathy is described with:**
     A   Subacute bacterial endocarditis
     B   Sjögren's syndrome
     C   Leishmaniasis
     D   Sarcoidosis
     E   Multiple myeloma

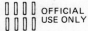

OFFICIAL USE ONLY

SURNAME	INITIALS
JOSHI	P

CANDIDATE NUMBER

THOU. 0 1 2 3 4 5 6 7 8 9

HUND. 0 1 2 3 4 5 6 7 8 9

| 4 | 7 | 5 | 6 |

TENS 0 1 2 3 4 5 6 7 8 9

UNITS 0 1 2 3 4 5 6 7 8 9

PAGE No.
1

T means TRUE F means FALSE D means DO NOT KNOW

20

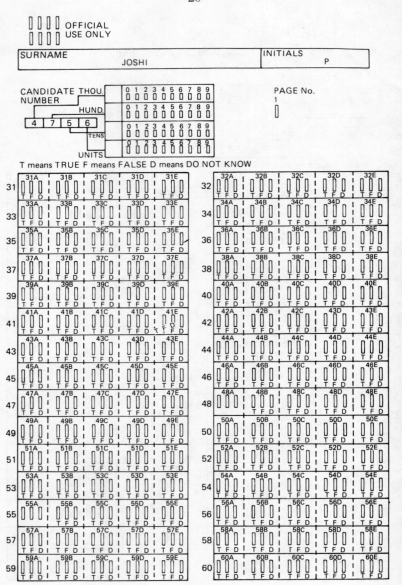

OFFICIAL USE ONLY

SURNAME	INITIALS
JOSHI	P

CANDIDATE NUMBER

THOU. 0 1 2 3 4 5 6 7 8 9
HUND. 0 1 2 3 4 5 6 7 8 9

4 7 5 6

TENS 0 1 2 3 4 5 6 7 8 9
UNITS 0 1 2 3 4 5 6 7 8 9

PAGE No.
1

T means TRUE F means FALSE D means DO NOT KNOW

Answers to Examination 1
(For complete References see Chapter 3)

1. A True (diuretic treatment, e.g. thiazides)
   B True
   C True
   D False (idiopathic in most cases)
   E False
   Ref. (1) pp. 126–138

2. A True (also true for allergic aspergillosis)
   B False (true for allergic/invasive aspergillosis)
   C True
   D True
   E False (characteristic of the allergic form)
   Ref. (2) pp. 742–743

3. A False (about 10%)
   B True
   C True
   D True
   E True
   Ref. (2) pp. 1896–1900

4. A True (produces exfoliative dermatitis)
   B False (methotrexate may be used in its treatment)
   C False
   D True
   E True
   Ref. (3) pp. 145–156

5. A True
   B False (with Addison's disease)
   C True
   D True
   E True
   Ref. (4) p. 68

6. A True
   B True
   C True
   D False
   E False (seen in primary or tertiary forms)
   Ref. (5) pp. 192–193

7. A True
   B True
   C True
   D True (may be on the fauces or tonsils)
   E True
   Ref. (2) pp. 801–804

8. A True
   B False
   C True
   D True (also penicillamine therapy)
   E False
   Ref. (6)

9. A False
   B False (foliate deficiency)
   C True
   D True
   E True
   Ref. (7) pp. 274–275

22

10. A   True
    B   False (autosomal
        recessive)
    C   False
    D   True
    E   True
    Ref. (8) pp. 425–426

11. A   False
    B   True
    C   True (commonest
        form of eye
        involvement)
    D   True
    E   False
    Ref. (1) pp. 114–119

12. A   True (portal
        hypertension
        following cirrhosis)
    B   False (chest
        infection)
    C   False
    D   True
    E   True
    Ref. (2) pp 1233–1235, 1511

13. A   True
    B   True
    C   True
    D   True
    E   True
    Ref. (4) pp. 299–300

14. A   True
    B   True
    C   True
    D   False
    E   False
    Ref. (2) pp. 876–879

15. A   True
    B   True
    C   False
    D   True
    E   False
    Ref. (9)

16. A   False (anaemia
        almost never severe)
    B   False (rare in
        children)
    C   True (rare in adults)
    D   True (because of
        increased intracranial
        pressure)
    E   True
    Ref. (2) pp. 967–968

17. A   False
    B   False
    C   True
    D   False
    E   True
    Ref. (6) pp. 433–434

18. A   True
    B   True
    C   False
    D   True
    E   False
    Ref. (2)

19. A   True
    B   True
    C   True
    D   True
    E   False
    Ref. (2) p. 2024

20. A   True
     B   True
     C   True (Austin Flint murmur)
     D   True (Carcy Coombs murmur)
     E   False
     Ref. (10)

21. A   True
     B   False (tall P waves—atrialization of right ventricle)
     C   True (Wolff–Parkinson–White syndrome type A)
     D   True
     E   True
     Ref. (11) pp. 35–36

22. A   True
     B   False (bladder function maintained until very late)
     C   True
     D   True
     E   False
     Ref. (8) pp. 1353–1354

23. A   True
     B   True
     C   False (leukoerythroblastic anaemia)
     D   False
     E   True (produces folate deficiency)
     Ref. (2) pp. 1518–1525

24. A   True
     B   False (used for its treatment)
     C   True
     D   False (used in its treatment; may produce nephrogenic diabetes insipidus)
     E   True (40% of all patients)
     Ref. (2) pp. 438–439, 1691–1694

25. A   False (due to any cause of hypercalcaemia)
     B   True
     C   False (any cause of hypercalcaemia)
     D   False (suggests non-metastatic hypercalcaemia)
     E   True (seen in primary hyper-parathyroidism)
     Ref. (2) pp. 1837–1838

26. A   True (directed against the I,i antigen system of the red cell)
     B   False (rare)
     C   False (seldom greater than 10% because anaemia is not severe)
     D   False
     E   True
     Ref. (2) pp. 1535–1537

27.   A   False (deep to the upper pole)
       B   True
       C   True (rare)
       D   True
       E   False (2nd–4th rings)
       Ref. (*14*) pp. 315–321

28.   A   True
       B   True
       C   True
       D   True
       E   False
       Ref. (*15*)

29.   A   True
       B   True
       C   False
       D   True
       E   False
       Ref. (*9*)

30.   A   False (infective only in the acute phase)
       B   True
       C   False
       D   True
       E   False
       Ref. (*2*) p. 881

31.   A   True
       B   True
       C   False
       D   False
       E   True
       Ref. (*2*) pp. 308–311

32.   A   True
       B   True
       C   False (young females)
       D   True
       E   False
       Ref. (*16*) p. 56

33.   A   False (hypocalcaemia)
       B   True
       C   False
       D   True
       E   True
       Ref. (*15*) pp. 67, 138, 140, 422, 443, 567

34.   A   True (normal up to 10)
       B   False
       C   False (greater than 130/ minute)
       D   False
       E   False
       Ref. (*9*) p. 127

35.   A   True
       B   False (assumes there is no significant difference)
       C   True
       D   True
       E   False (is the mode)
       Ref. (*17*)

36.   A   False
       B   True
       C   False (hyper-parathyroidism)
       D   True
       E   True
       Ref. (*2*) pp. 1371–1384

37.   A   False
       B   False
       C   False
       D   True
       E   False (found in infective endocarditis)
       Ref. (*18*) p. 31
            (*10*) pp. 364–370

38. A   False (reactive
         depression)
     B   False (early-morning
         waking)
     C   True
     D   False (slow response;
         therefore, if severe,
         electroconvulsive
         therapy is the
         treatment of choice)
     E   False
     Ref. (*19*) pp. 439–476

39. A   False
     B   True (of low sugar
         content)
     C   True
     D   True
     E   True
     Ref. (*1*) pp. 35–41

40. A   False (secondary
         biliary cirrhosis)
     B   True (a frequent
         finding)
     C   True
     D   True
     E   False
     Ref. (*8*) p. 654

41. A   True
     B   False
     C   True
     D   True
     E   False
     Ref. (*6*)

42. A   False
     B   False
     C   True
     D   False (related to
         radiation therapy)
     E   True
     Ref. (*1*) pp. 107–114

43. A   True
     B   True (if uncontrolled
         hyperglycaemia, or
         in the presence of
         acidosis)
     C   False
     D   False
     E   True
     Ref. (*5*) pp. 27–28

44. A   True
     B   False
         (hypoglycaemia)
     C   False
     D   True
     E   True
     Ref. (*2*)

45. A   False
     B   True
     C   True
     D   True
     E   False
     Ref. (*6*) p. 719

46. A   False (4th day)
     B   True
     C   True
     D   False
     E   False
     Ref. (*8*)

47. A   True
     B   False
     C   True
     D   True
     E   False
     Ref. (*2*) pp. 805–806

48. A   False
     B   False
     C   True
     D   True
     E   True
     Ref. (*20*) pp. 6–7

49. A True
    B True
    C True
    D False
    E False
    Ref. (*2*) p. 202

50. A False (hypertrophic
         obstructive
         cardiomyopathy—
         HOCM)
    B True
    C False (HOCM)
    D True
    E False (HOCM)
    Ref. (*10*) pp. 435–445

51. A False
         (dexamphetamines)
    B True (in 60% of
         cases)
    C False
    D True
    E True
    Ref. (*2*) p. 129

52. A True
    B False
    C False
    D True
    E True
    Ref. (*6*)

53. A False (temporal lobe
         epilepsy)
    B False (acute
         glaucoma)
    C False (Todd's
         paralysis implies
         localization)
    D True (petit mal
         epilepsy)
    E True (occurs only in
         a small number of
         patients)
    Ref. (*8*) pp. 1245–1247

54. A False (Epanutin
         therapy)
    B True
    C False
    D True
    E True
    Ref. (*2*)

55. A True (even without
         underlying
         neoplasm)
    B False (mid and lower
         zones affected)
    C True
    D True
    E False
    Ref. (*8*) pp. 592, 906–907

56. A False
    B True (asterixis)
    C True
    D True
    E True
    Ref. (*2*) pp. 1459–1472

57. A True
    B False
    C True
    D False
    E True
    Ref. (*21*) p. 544
         (*5*) pp. 3–5

58. A True
    B True
    C False
    D True
    E False
    Ref. (*2*)

59. A False
    B True
    C False
    D True
    E True
    Ref. (*20*) pp. 22–23

60. A   True
    B   True
    C   True
    D   True
    E   False (monoclonal
              gammopathy)
    Ref. (*4*)

Examination 2

(Time allotted: 2½ hours)

1. **A small pulse pressure is characteristic of:**
   A Patent ductus arteriosus
   B Aortic stenosis
   C Severe pulmonary stenosis
   D Shoshin beriberi heart disease
   E Mitral stenosis

2. **Typical features of neurofibromatosis include:**
   A Bony abnormalities
   B Plexiform neuromata
   C Photophobia
   D Pachydermoperiostitis
   E Paroxysmal hypertension occurring infrequently

3. **In carpal tunnel syndrome:**
   A Tapping over the ulnar nerve reproduces symptoms
   B It may be precipitated by pregnancy
   C Steroid therapy is urgently indicated
   D Myxoedema may be associated
   E Wasting of the hypothenar muscles is characteristic

4. **Injury to the occipital cortex results in:**
   A Homonymous hemianopia
   B Loss of central field of vision
   C Altitudinal hemianopia
   D Pupillary changes
   E Organized visual hallucinations

5. **Neurotic obsession is characterized by:**
   A   Repetitive behaviour
   B   Relief of distress and anxiety
   C   Escape from unpleasant situation
   D   The patient regards it as abnormal
   E   The patient seeks to attract attention

6. **Sacroiliitis is a feature of:**
   A   Gout
   B   Sarcoidosis
   C   Reiter's syndrome
   D   Psoriatic arthritis
   E   Ankylosing spondylitis

7. **Dupuytren's contractures are typically associated with:**
   A   Epilepsy
   B   Alcoholic hepatic cirrhosis
   C   Chronic rheumatoid arthritis
   D   Diabetes mellitus
   E   Shoulder-hand syndrome

8. **In Wilson's disease:**
   A   Kaiser–Fleisher rings remain following therapy
   B   Chondrocalcinosis is described
   C   Basal ganglia calcification results
   D   Fanconi's syndrome may occur
   E   A wing-beating flap is characteristic

9. **Recognized treatment of alcohol-induced acute pancreatitis includes:**
   A   Intravenous fluid administration and nasogastric suction
   B   Prophylactic ampicillin
   C   Peritoneal lavage
   D   Intravenous hydrocortisone
   E   Correction of hypercalcaemia

10. **Treatment of diabetes insipidus includes:**
    A   Chlorpropamide
    B   Clorexolone (Nefrolan)
    C   Synthetic lysine vasopressin
    D   Thiazide diuretics
    E   Subcutaneous insulin

11. **Koebner's phenomenon is demonstrable in:**
    A   Reiter's syndrome
    B   Lichen planus
    C   Mycosis fungoides
    D   Psoriasis
    E   Pityriasis rosea

12. **The following should be avoided in patients on monoamine oxidase inhibitor therapy:**
    A   Cheese
    B   Tofranil
    C   Phentolamine
    D   Pethidine
    E   Sulphonamides

13. **In Klinefelter's syndrome:**
    A   47 XXY chromosomal pattern is found
    B   Patients have small, soft testes
    C   Gynaecomastia is common
    D   Patent ductus arteriosus is associated
    E   An association with diabetes mellitus exists

14. **Erythema nodosum is well recognized with:**
    A   Rheumatoid arthritis
    B   Crohn's disease
    C   Post-streptococcal infection
    D   Contraceptive pill usage
    E   Meningococcal meningitis

15. **Rash on the palms and soles is seen in:**
    A   Pompholyx
    B   Secondary syphilis
    C   Chicken pox
    D   Erythema gyratum perstans
    E   Guttate form of psoriasis

16. **The following features differentiate sarcoidosis from berylliosis:**
    A Uveitis
    B Chest x-ray appearances
    C Erythema nodosum
    D Mantoux test
    E Lupus pernio

17. **Antinuclear factor is typically negative in:**
    A Rheumatoid arthritis
    B Dermatomyositis
    C Scleroderma
    D Polyarteritis nodosa
    E Infective endocarditis

18. **Paroxysmal nocturnal haemoglobinuria:**
    A Is associated with chronic intravascular haemolysis
    B Is associated with haemosiderinuria
    C May present with repeated venous thromboses
    D May transform to chronic myeloid leukaemia
    E Chloroquin is contraindicated

19. **The following factors decrease gastric emptying:**
    A High protein meal
    B Ingestion of ferrous gluconate
    C Acidity in the duodenum
    D Vagal stimulation
    E Alcohol ingestion

20. **Infectious mononucleosis (glandular fever):**
    A Produces splenomegaly in all patients
    B May be related to Epstein–Barr virus
    C Requires a lymph node biopsy for the diagnosis
    D Can be diagnosed on the Weil–Felix reaction
    E Produces a rash following Ampicillin in over 90% of cases

21. **Tunnel vision is seen with:**
   A   Vitamin A deficiency
   B   Acute glaucoma
   C   Papilloedema
   D   Exophthalmic ophthalmoplegia
   E   Hysteria

22. **Creatinine phosphokinase levels are elevated:**
   A   24 hours postmyocardial infarction
   B   In thyrotoxicosis
   C   In polymyositis
   D   In polymyalgia rheumatica
   E   In a severe asthmatic attack

23. **The following drugs may produce the nephrotic syndrome:**
   A   Epanutin
   B   Colchicine
   C   Penicillamine
   D   Troxidone
   E   Mercurials

24. **In anorexia nervosa:**
   A   Gonadotrophin deficiency is found
   B   Muscle weakness may be related to hypokalaemia
   C   The patients are characteristically hyperactive
   D   Response to medical treatment is excellent
   E   There is a high incidence of suicide

25. **Conn's syndrome is characterized by:**
   A   A raised serum sodium
   B   A raised urinary potassium
   C   Circumoral parasthesiae
   D   Tendency to develop malignant hypertension
   E   Severe peripheral pedal oedema

26. **Causes of renal papillar necrosis include:**
   A   Sickle–cell disease
   B   Salicylate therapy
   C   Macroglobulinaemia
   D   Outdated tetracycline therapy
   E   Diabetes mellitus

27. **Side-effects of streptomycin are:**
   A   Enhanced by associated folate deficiency
   B   Production of irreversible vestibular damage
   C   Liable to occur with chronic liver disease
   D   Not seen if the drug is given orally
   E   More common in the elderly

28. **Acute pancreatitis is known to cause:**
   A   Obstructive jaundice
   B   Hyperglycaemia
   C   Hyponatremia
   D   Tender lesions on the shins
   E   A decrease in the Pa_{O_2}

29. **In primary biliary cirrhosis:**
   A   Hepatomegaly is commonly tender
   B   Severe itching may precede clinical jaundice
   C   Splenomegaly is usually present
   D   Ascites is a common early feature
   E   There is a high association with renal tubular acidosis

30. **Drugs producing jaundice include:**
   A   Phenobarbitones
   B   Hydrallazine
   C   Diazoxide
   D   Chlorpropamide
   E   Chlorpromazine

31. **Typical features of complete heart block are:**
   A   A wide pulse pressure
   B   Irregular cannon 'a' waves
   C   Paradoxical splitting of the second heart sound
   D   Increase in pulse rate with amyl nitrite
   E   Mid–diastolic murmur over the apex

32. **A false positive Albustix text is produced in:**
   A   Fevers
   B   Infected urine
   C   Ulcerative colitis
   D   Pregnancy
   E   Presence of mucoprotein

33. **The following symptoms may be found in a patient with renal tubular acidosis:**
    A   Muscle cramps
    B   Loin pain on micturition
    C   Constipation
    D   Dizziness on standing up suddenly
    E   Back pain

34. **Catatonic schizophrenia:**
    A   Characteristically affects the 45–55-year age group
    B   Is commoner in males
    C   In the stupor form typically produces amnesia
    D   Commonly produces vasomotor disturbances
    E   Requires electroconvulsive therapy as the treatment of choice if severe stupor is present

35. **The following statements are true regarding coeliac disease:**
    A   It usually begins in the first three years of life
    B   The patient may be allowed to eat oats
    C   Characteristic changes are seen in the gastric mucosa
    D   Steroids must be given in high doses
    E   There is an increased incidence of intestinal lymphoma

36. **Prolongation of the Q–T interval is seen in:**
    A   Hypocalcaemia
    B   Pericardial effusion
    C   Acute rheumatic fever
    D   Severe aortic stenosis
    E   Procainamide therapy

37. **A patient with osteomalacia due to the Malabsorption syndrome may present with:**
    A   A waddling gait
    B   Difficulty in climbing stairs
    C   Looser's zones seen on x-ray of the pelvis
    D   Production of generalized lymphadenopathy as a rule
    E   A high mortality without treatment

38. **Dengue:**
   A   Is produced by an arbovirus
   B   Is transmitted by the sandfly
   C   Commonly produces severe retro-orbital pain
   D   Generalized lymphadenopathy is the rule
   E   Mortality is high without treatment

39. **Rigors are characteristic of:**
   A   Rubella
   B   Sarcoidosis
   C   Secondary syphilis
   D   Ascending cholangitis
   E   Falciparum malaria

40. **Albright's disease (fibrous dysplasia) typically produces:**
   A   Osteitis fibrosa disseminata
   B   Low output failure
   C   Pigmentation
   D   Precocious puberty
   E   Convulsions

41. **In the following, inheritance is autosomal dominant:**
   A   Haemophilia
   B   Von Willebrand's disease
   C   Phenylketonuria
   D   Duchenne's pseudohypertrophic muscular dystrophy
   E   Adult form of polycystic kidneys

42. **The following anatomical data are true:**
   A   Opponens pollicis muscle is innervated by the ulnar nerve
   B   Abductor pollicis brevis is supplied by the median nerve
   C   The diaphragm is innervated by C3, 4 and 5
   D   Lower cord of the brachial plexus comprises C8, T1 and 2
   E   The knee jerk is innervated by L3 and 4 segments

43. **Pulmonary diffusion defects are described in:**
    A   Acute pneumonia
    B   Inhalation of a foreign body
    C   Alveolar-cell carcinoma
    D   Acute pulmonary oedema
    E   Guillain–Barré syndrome

44. **Scleroderma (systemic sclerosis) may be associated with:**
    A   Recurrent chest infections
    B   Restrictive lung defect on pulmonary function testing
    C   Wheezing
    D   Alveolar-cell carcinoma
    E   Oesophageal varices

45. **The following may produce secondary polycythaemia:**
    A   Cushing's syndrome
    B   Uterine myomata
    C   Primary hepatoma
    D   Gastric carcinoma
    E   Cerebellar gumma

46. **Skin lesions associated with bronchogenic carcinoma include:**
    A   Erythema gyratum perstans
    B   Pityriasis rosea
    C   Acanthosis nigricans
    D   Pompholyx
    E   Erythroderma

47. **Gonococcal septicaemia may produce:**
    A   Polyarthritis
    B   A hepatic friction rub
    C   Endocarditis
    D   Spontaneous splenic rupture
    E   A haemorrhagic skin rash

48. **Phenylketonuria produces:**
    A   Mental retardation
    B   Photosensitivity
    C   Convulsions
    D   Death by the age of five years
    E   Associated atrial septal defect

49. **The causes of hepatosplenomegaly in a ten-year-old child include:**
    A   Gaucher's disease
    B   Medulloblastoma with metastatic spread
    C   Leukaemia
    D   Primary biliary cirrhosis
    E   Congenital rubella syndrome

50. **Herpes zoster:**
    A   Commonly affects the ophthalmic division of the fifth nerve
    B   Is due to the chicken pox virus
    C   Should be treated with idoxuridine
    D   Rash may be preceded by severe pain in the affected site
    E   Produces post-herpetic neuralgia as a distressing complication

51. **Cocaine addiction—the following statements are true:**
    A   Commonly produces pruritis
    B   Is associated with marked dependence
    C   Greater than 90% of addicts have underlying psychiatric disturbances
    D   It is seen most frequently in adolescents
    E   Tolerance is related to the ability of the kidney to excrete it

52. **Acromegaly is commonly associated with:**
    A   Thickening of the heel pad
    B   Homonymous hemianopia
    C   Hyperostosis frontalis
    D   Hypoglycaemia
    E   Increased sweating

53. **Increased cerebrospinal fluid globulins are seen in:**
   A Motor neurone disease
   B Guillain–Barré syndrome
   C Subacute sclerosing panencephalitis
   D Parkinson's disease
   E Disseminated sclerosis

54. **Pulsus paradoxus may be found with:**
   A A severe asthmatic attack
   B Severe left ventricular failure
   C A flabby myocardium
   D Constrictive pericarditis
   E Cardiac amyloidosis

55. **Massive haemoptysis is a well recognized feature of:**
   A Carcinoma of the bronchus
   B Goodpasture's syndrome
   C Acute pulmonary oedema
   D Bleeding Rasmussen's aneurysm in tuberculosis
   E Pneumococcal lobar pneumonia

56. **The following conditions cause pancytopenia:**
   A Blackfan–Diamond syndrome
   B Addisonian pernicious anaemia
   C Paroxysmal nocturnal haemoglobinuria
   D Hypersplenism
   E Chronic disseminated intravascular coagulation

57. **Korsakoff's psychosis may be caused by:**
   A Marihuana smoking
   B Carbon monoxide poisoning
   C Vitamin B deficiency
   D Uncontrolled diabetes mellitus
   E Lead poisoning

58. **Recognized causes of malabsorption include:**
   A Systemic sclerosis
   B Ileal lymphoma
   C Atherosclerosis of the superior mesenteric artery
   D Amoebiasis
   E Jejunal diverticulosis

59. **Perforating ulcers of the foot may occur in:**
   A   Varicose veins
   B   Sickle–cell disease
   C   Tuberculoid leprosy
   D   Diabetes mellitus
   E   Lead neuropathy

60. **In the chi–square test:**
   A   Chi–square value is always equal to or greater than 0
   B   The Null hypothesis is used
   C   The greater the value of chi–square, the less likely it is to be significant
   D   Only pilot studies may be evaluated
   E   Overall difference between observed and expected frequencies is measured

OFFICIAL USE ONLY

SURNAME	INITIALS
JOSHI	P

CANDIDATE NUMBER: 4 7 5 6

THOU.	0 1 2 3 4 5 6 7 8 9
HUND.	0 1 2 3 4 5 6 7 8 9
TENS	0 1 2 3 4 5 6 7 8 9
UNITS	0 1 2 3 4 5 6 7 8 9

PAGE No. 1

T means TRUE F means FALSE D means DO NOT KNOW

1	1A T F D	1B T F D	1C T F D	1D T F D	1E T F D
3	3A T F D	3B T F D	3C T F D	3D T F D	3E T F D
5	5A T F D	5B T F D	5C T F D	5D T F D	5E T F D
7	7A T F D	7B T F D	7C T F D	7D T F D	7E T F D
9	9A T F D	9B T F D	9C T F D	9D T F D	9E T F D
11	11A T F D	11B T F D	11C T F D	11D T F D	11E T F D
13	13A T F D	13B T F D	13C T F D	13D T F D	13E T F D
15	15A T F D	15B T F D	15C T F D	15D T F D	15E T F D
17	17A T F D	17B T F D	17C T F D	17D T F D	17E T F D
19	19A T F D	19B T F D	19C T F D	19D T F D	19E T F D
21	21A T F D	21B T F D	21C T F D	21D T F D	21E T F D
23	23A T F D	23B T F D	23D T F D	23C T F D	23E T F D
25	25A T F D	25B T F D	25C T F D	25D T F D	25E T F D
27	27A T F D	27B T F D	27C T F D	27D T F D	27E T F D
29	29A T F D	29B T F D	29C T F D	29D T F D	29E T F D

2	2A T F D	2B T F D	2C T F D	2D T F D	2E T F D
4	4A T F D	4B T F D	4C T F D	4D T F D	4E T F D
6	6A T F D	6B T F D	6C T F D	6D T F D	6E T F D
8	8A T F D	8B T F D	8C T F D	8D T F D	8E T F D
10	10A T F D	10B T F D	10C T F D	10D T F D	10E T F D
12	12A T F D	12B T F D	12C T F D	12D T F D	12E T F D
14	14A T F D	14B T F D	14C T F D	14D T F D	14E T F D
16	16A T F D	16B T F D	16C T F D	16D T F D	16E T F D
18	18A T F D	18B T F D	18C T F D	18D T F D	18E T F D
20	20A T F D	20B T F D	20C T F D	20D T F D	20E T F D
22	22A T F D	22B T F D	22C T F D	22D T F D	22E T F D
24	24A T F D	24B T F D	24C T F D	24D T F D	24E T F D
26	26A T F D	26B T F D	26C T F D	26D T F D	26E T F D
28	28A T F D	28B T F D	28C T F D	28D T F D	28E T F D
30	30A T F D	30B T F D	30C T F D	30D T F D	30E T F D

OFFICIAL USE ONLY

SURNAME	INITIALS
JOSHI	P

CANDIDATE NUMBER

THOU. 0 1 2 3 4 5 6 7 8 9

HUND. 0 1 2 3 4 5 6 7 8 9

| 4 | 7 | 5 | 6 |

TENS 0 1 2 3 4 5 6 7 8 9

UNITS 0 1 2 3 4 5 6 7 8 9

PAGE No.
1

T means TRUE F means FALSE D means DO NOT KNOW

31	31A T F D	31B T F D	31C T F D	31D T F D	31E T F D
33	33A T F D	33B T F D	33C T F D	33D T F D	33E T F D
35	35A T F D	35B T F D	35C T F D	35D T F D	35E T F D
37	37A T F D	37B T F D	37C T F D	37D T F D	37E T F D
39	39A T F D	39B T F D	39C T F D	39D T F D	39E T F D
41	41A T F D	41B T F D	41C T F D	41D T F D	41E T F D
43	43A T F D	43B T F D	43C T F D	43D T F D	43E T F D
45	45A T F D	45B T F D	45C T F D	45D T F D	45E T F D
47	47A T F D	47B T F D	47C T F D	47D T F D	47E T F D
49	49A T F D	49B T F D	49C T F D	49D T F D	49E T F D
51	51A T F D	51B T F D	51C T F D	51D T F D	51E T F D
53	53A T F D	53B T F D	53C T F D	53D T F D	53E T F D
55	55A T F D	55B T F D	55C T F D	55D T F D	55E T F D
57	57A T F D	57B T F D	57C T F D	57D T F D	57E T F D
59	59A T F D	59B T F D	59C T F D	59D T F D	59E T F D

32	32A T F D	32B T F D	32C T F D	32D T F D	32E T F D
34	34A T F D	34B T F D	34C T F D	34D T F D	34E T F D
36	36A T F D	36B T F D	36C T F D	36D T F D	36E T F D
38	38A T F D	38B T F D	38C T F D	38D T F D	38E T F D
40	40A T F D	40B T F D	40C T F D	40D T F D	40E T F D
42	42A T F D	42B T F D	42C T F D	43D T F D	43E T F D
44	44A T F D	44B T F D	44C T F D	44D T F D	44E T F D
46	46A T F D	46B T F D	46C T F D	46D T F D	46E T F D
48	48A T F D	48B T F D	48C T F D	48D T F D	48E T F D
50	50A T F D	50B T F D	50C T F D	50D T F D	50E T F D
52	52A T F D	52B T F D	52C T F D	52D T F D	52E T F D
54	54A T F D	54B T F D	54C T F D	54D T F D	54E T F D
56	56A T F D	56B T F D	56C T F D	56D T F D	56E T F D
58	58A T F D	58B T F D	58C T F D	58D T F D	58E T F D
60	60A T F D	60B T F D	60C T F D	60D T F D	60E T F D

Answers to Examination 2
(For complete References see Chapter 3)

1.   A   False (collapsing
              pulse)
     B   True
     C   True
     D   True (associated
              with shock)
     E   True
     Ref. (10) pp. 26–27

2.   A   True
     B   True
     C   False
     D   False
     E   True (associated
              phaeochromo-
              cytoma)
     Ref. (2) pp. 2006–2007

3.   A   False (median nerve)
     B   True
     C   False
     D   True
     E   False (thenar
              muscles)
     Ref. (2) p. 1903

4.   A   True
     B   True
     C   True
     D   False
     E   True
     Ref. (2) p. 147

5.   A   True
     B   True
     C   False
     D   True
     E   False
     Ref. (2) pp. 71, 73

6.   A   False
     B   False
     C   True
     D   True
     E   True
     Ref. (1)

7.   A   True
     B   True
     C   False
     D   True
     E   False
     Ref. (20) pp. 31, 35, 39, 200

8.   A   False
     B   True
     C   False (in
              hypocalcaemia)
     D   True
     E   True
     Ref. (8) pp. 572–573, 1363

9.   A   True
     B   False
     C   True
     D   False
     E   False
              (hypocalcaemia)
     Ref. (2) pp. 1503–1511

10.   A   True
     B   True
     C   True
     D   True
     E   False
     Ref. (8) pp. 488–489

11. A   False
    B   True
    C   False
    D   True
    E   False
    Ref. (*3*) p. 36

12. A   True
    B   True
    C   False (reverses
          hypertensive effect)
    D   True
    E   False
    Ref. (*7*) pp. 268–270

13. A   True
    B   False (firm testes)
    C   True
    D   False
    E   True
    Ref. (*3*) pp. 104, 111

14. A   False
    B   True
    C   True
    D   True
    E   False
    Ref. (*3*) p. 128

15. A   True
    B   True
    C   False
    D   False
    E   False
    Ref. (*8*) See section on
    Dermatology. You must
    know the causes of
    papular eruptions,
    pustular eruptions,
    bullous lesions, etc.

16. A   True
    B   False
    C   True
    D   False
    E   True
    Ref. (*2*) pp. 928–932, 1219,
    1220

17. A   False
    B   True
    C   False
    D   True
    E   False
    Ref. (*8*)

18. A   True
    B   True
    C   True
    D   False (myeloblastic
          leukaemia)
    E   False
    Ref. (*2*) pp. 1540–1541

19. A   False (fatty meal)
    B   False
    C   True
    D   False (vagotomy
          does)
    E   False
    Ref. (*21*) p. 380

20. A   False (about 30%)
    B   True
    C   False (Paul-Bunnel
          test)
    D   False (as above in C)
    E   True
    Ref. (*2*) pp. 854–857

21. A False
        (hypervitaminosis A
        may produce
        papilloedema)
     B True
     C True
     D False
     E True
     Ref. (23) pp. 19–20
           (2) p. 104
     Look up disturbances of
     vision in the references
     given here.

22. A True
     B False
        (hypothyroidism)
     C True
     D False
     E True
     Ref. (4) p. 40

23. A False
     B False
     C True
     D True
     E True
     Ref. (5) p. 73

24. A True
     B True
     C True
     D False (may be very
        difficult to treat)
     E False
     Ref. (2) pp. 416–418

25. A True
     B True
     C True (hypokalaemic
        alkalosis produces
        hypocalcaemia)
     D False (very unusual)
     E False
     Ref. (16) p. 38

26. A True
     B False
     C True
     D False
     E True
     Ref. (5) pp. 34–36

27. A False
     B True
     C False (with renal
        disease)
     D True (because of
        poor absorption)
     E True (especially if
        associated renal
        insufficiency)
     Ref. (7) pp. 482–483

28. A True (oedema of the
        head of the pancreas)
     B True
     C False
        (hypocalcaemia)
     D True (metastatic fat
        necrosis)
     E True
     Ref. (2) pp. 1503–1507

29. A True
     B True
     C True (because of
        portal hypertension)
     D False (hepatic
        function preserved
        until late)
     E True
     Ref. (2) pp. 1476, 1478

30. A False
     B False
     C False
     D True
     E True
     Ref. (18) p. 190

31.
A   True
B   True
C   False
D   False
E   False
Ref. (*10*) pp. 210, 213–218

32.
A   False
B   True
C   False
D   True
E   True
Ref. (*8*) pp. 1000–1001

33.
A   True (hypokalaemia)
B   True (nephrolithiasis)
C   False
D   False
E   True (osteomalacia)
Ref. (*5*) pp. 149–152

34.
A   False (about 25 years)
B   False (females)
C   False
D   True
E   True
Ref. (*19*) pp. 405–407

35.
A   True
B   True
C   False (jejunum)
D   False
E   True
Ref. (*8*) 641–642)

36.
A   True
B   False
C   True
D   False
E   True
Ref. (*11*) p. 143. Also true for:
Diffuse myocardial disease
Myocardial infarction
Cerebrovascular accident
Head injury
Quinidine effect
Cardiac syncope

37.
A   True
B   True
C   True
D   False
E   False
Ref. (*16*) p. 153

38.
A   True
B   False (Aëdes aegypti mosquito)
C   True
D   False
E   False (mortality is nil)
Ref. (*2*) pp. 829–830

39.
A   False
B   False
C   False
D   True
E   True
Ref. (*24*) p. 50

40.
A   True
B   False (increased cardiac output found)
C   True
D   True
E   False
Ref. (*8*) pp. 979–980

41.
A False
B True
C False
D False
E True
Ref. (*25*) p. 1007

42.
A False (median nerve)
B True
C True
D False (C8, T1)
E True
Ref. (*14*) pp. 16, 233–234

43.
A True
B False
C True
D True
E False
Ref. (*9*)

44.
A True
B True
C False
D True (very rarely; also true for bronchiolar cell carcinoma)
E False
Ref. (*2*) pp. 1896–1900

45.
A True
B True
C True
D False
E False
Ref. (*8*) p. 1189

46.
A True
B False
C True
D False
E True
Ref. (*8*) p. 897

47.
A True
B True (owing to a perihepatitis)
C True
D False
E True
Ref. (*2*) pp. 624–629

48.
A True
B True
C True
D False
E False
Ref. (*8*) pp. 425–426

49.
A True
B False
C True
D False
E False
Ref. (*15*)

50.
A True
B True
C False
D True
E True
Ref. (*2*) pp. 801–804

51.
A True
B False
C True
D True
E False
Ref. (*19*) pp. 676–677
(*35*) p. 229

52.
A True
B False (bitemporal hemianopia)
C False
D False (hyperglycaemia)
E True
Ref. (*16*) p. 5

53. A   False
    B   True
    C   True
    D   False
    E   True
    Ref. (4) pp. 172–175

54. A   True
    B   False
    C   True
    D   True
    E   True
    Ref. (10) pp. 31–32

55. A   True
    B   True
    C   False
    D   True
    E   False
    Ref. (9) pp. 30, 263

56. A   False (pure red-cell
          aplasia)
    B   True
    C   True
    D   True
    E   False
    Ref. (4) p. 211

57. A   False
    B   True
    C   True
    D   False
    E   True
    Ref. (2) p. 149

58. A   True
    B   True
    C   True
    D   False
    E   True
    Ref. (2) pp. 1396–1409

59. A   False
    B   False
    C   True
    D   True
    E   False (motor
          neuropathy)
    Ref. (2) pp. 243–244

60. A   True
    B   True
    C   False (more likely)
    D   False
    E   True
    Ref. (17)

Examination 3

(Time allotted: 2½ hours)

1. **Well recognized causes of erythema multiforme include:**
   A Contraceptive pill
   B Herpes simplex infection
   C Underlying malignancy
   D Mycoplasma pneumonia
   E Pemphigus foliaceus

2. **Acute hypercalcaemia may be treated with:**
   A Sodium phosphate solution intramuscularly
   B Mithramycin
   C Bromocriptine
   D Calcitonin
   E Furosemide intravenously

3. **In Henoch–Schönlein purpura:**
   A Thrombocytopenia is common
   B Small bowel intussusception may occur
   C Presentation may be similar to acute nephritis
   D 30% develop progressive glomerulonephritis
   E A rash confined to the shoulders is commonly produced

4. **Chronic active hepatitis is described with:**
   A   Ulcerative colitis
   B   Alpha-methyldopa therapy
   C   Oxyphenisatin usage
   D   Wilson's disease
   E   Alpha-1-antitrypsin deficiency

5. **Ehlers–Danlos syndrome may be associated with:**
   A   Dissecting aneurysm of the aorta
   B   Recurrent pneumothoraces
   C   Diaphragmatic hernia
   D   Coarctation of the aorta
   E   Diverticuli of the gastrointestinal tract

6. **The following features support the diagnosis of a polymyositis in preference to a muscular dystrophy:**
   A   Non-selective weakness
   B   Presence of hypertrophy of muscles
   C   Weakness out of proportion to muscle wasting
   D   Raynaud's phenomenon
   E   Early finding of absent reflexes

7. **Characteristic features of sickle-cell anaemia are:**
   A   Painful swollen fingers
   B   Aseptic necrosis of the femoral head
   C   Howell–Jolly bodies on blood smear in adults
   D   Higher incidence of Down's syndrome (Mongolism)
   E   Improvement of symptoms at high altitudes

8. **Recognized causes of pruritis include:**
   A   Acromegaly
   B   Hypoparathyroidism
   C   Polycythaemia rubra vera
   D   Pernicious anaemia
   E   Hodgkin's lymphoma

9. **The following features are commonly found in systemic lupus erythematosis:**

A Temporomandibular joint involvement
B Systemic hypertension
C Mitral incompetence
D Central nervous system involvement
E Non-deforming polyarthritis

10. **Arthritis in ulcerative colitis:**

A Mainly affects small joints
B May present a syndrome similar to ankylosing spondylitis
C Is invariable when iritis is present
D Is an indication for steroid therapy
E Usually remits after colectomy

11. **The following statements are true regarding acute myocardial infarction:**

A It may be produced by severe tachyarrhythmias
B Thrombotic occlusion of the coronary artery is found in up to 85% in postmortem studies
C Patients are more prone to develop attacks in the winter months than in summer
D If the acute pain comes on at rest, the diagnosis of myocardial infarction is unlikely
E In old healed infarcts clearcut evidence on the electrocardiogram is found in less than one-third of patients

12. **Methotrexate administered intrathecally may produce:**

A Dryness of the mouth
B Raised intracranial pressure
C Folic acid deficiency
D Cranial nerve palsy
E Headaches

13. **The following drugs have proven value in the treatment of multiple myeloma:**
   A   Sodium fluoride
   B   Corticosteroids
   C   Regular doses of alkali
   D   Diphenylhydantoin
   E   Melphalan

14. **The following statements regarding Q fever are true:**
   A   It may produce infective endocarditis
   B   It is acquired by drinking unpasteurized milk
   C   It is commoner in females
   D   Penicillin in high doses is the treatment of choice
   E   The prognosis with treatment is excellent

15. **The following are features of an atrial myxoma:**
   A   Commonest site is the right atrium
   B   May present with recurrent pulmonary oedema
   C   The development of pulmonary hypertension
   D   Typical elevation of the gamma globulins
   E   Shows classical electrocardiographic changes

16. **Von Willebrand's disease is characterized by:**
   A   Autosomal recessive inheritance
   B   Factor VIII deficiency
   C   Thrombocytopenia
   D   Unresponsiveness to cryoprecipitate administration
   E   Prolonged bleeding time

17. **In primary pulmonary hypertension the following are true:**
   A   Recurrent syncopal attacks occur
   B   Dull retrosternal chest pain occurs
   C   Raised pulmonary capillary wedge pressure is found
   D   Left anterior hemiblock is seen on the electrocardiogram
   E   Raynaud's phenomenon occurs

18. **Antimitochondrial antibodies are found in:**
   A Cryptogenic cirrhosis
   B Contraceptive pill users
   C Chronic active hepatitis
   D Primary hepatocellular carcinoma
   E Primary biliary cirrhosis

19. **Bromocriptine is of value in the treatment of:**
   A Severe asthma
   B Hyperprolactinaemia
   C Secondary infertility
   D Acromegaly
   E Parkinson's syndrome

20. **Psoriatic joint involvement includes:**
   A Rheumatoid-like arthritis
   B Higher incidence of septic arthritis
   C Sacroiliitis'
   D Temporomandibular joint involvement
   E Arthritis mutilans

21. **In the cholinergic crisis associated with the treatment of myasthenia gravis, the following are true:**
   A Results from excessive atropine therapy
   B Fasciculations occur
   C Dysarthria may result
   D Mydriasis occurs
   E Intravenous Tensilon (edrophonium) produces worsening of symptoms

22. **The following are typical features of neurogenic pulmonary oedema:**
   A It is frequently related to lesions affecting the hypothalamus
   B May follow non-penetrating head injury
   C The protein content of the pulmonary oedema fluid is less than 25g/litre (2.5g%)
   D It is prevented by giving adrenergic drugs
   E Radiographic appearances are indistinguishable from other causes of pulmonary oedema

23. **Behçet's disease is characterized by:**
   A   Deforming polyarthritis
   B   Relapsing iritis
   C   Hepatosplenomegaly
   D   Painful orogenital ulcers
   E   Common occurrence of erythema nodosum

24. **The following are true regarding ventricular aneurysms:**
   A   Presence of 3rd and 4th heart sounds is diagnostic
   B   Always undergoes calcification
   C   More likely to occur with full thickness myocardial infarction
   D   Produces characteristic electrocardiographic changes
   E   May produce persistent angina

25. **Purpura may be produced with:**
   A   Henoch–Schönlein syndrome
   B   Cirrhosis of the liver
   C   Systemic lupus erythematosus
   D   Addison's disease
   E   Raynaud's phenomenon

26. **In Horner's syndrome:**
   A   Complete ptosis is usual
   B   The pupil is usually dilated
   C   Sweating is increased on the affected side
   D   Posterior communicating artery aneurysm is a well-recognized cause
   E   May be produced by diabetes mellitus

27. **Digoxin toxicity may produce:**
   A   Trigeminal neuralgia
   B   Red–green colour blindness
   C   Paroxysmal atrial tachycardia with atrioventricular block
   D   Bundle-branch block
   E   Bidirectional ventricular tachycardia

28. **Bone density is significantly increased in:**
   A   Osteopetrosis (marble bone disease)
   B   Paget's disease of bone
   C   Ingestion of fluorides in large amounts
   D   Hyperparathyroidism
   E   Renal osteodystrophy

29. **Acute pancreatitis may be associated with:**
   A   Biliary tract disease
   B   Furosemide therapy
   C   Hyperthyroidism
   D   Hypocalcaemia
   E   Type IIa hypercholesterolaemia

30. **The following symptoms are important in the clinical staging of Hodgkin's disease:**
   A   Greater than 10% loss of weight within six months
   B   Pruritis
   C   Pyrexia of unknown aetiology
   D   Alcohol intolerance
   E   Nocturnal sweats

31. **Pleural calcification is seen with:**
   A   Severe mitral stenosis
   B   Miliary tuberculosis
   C   Cryptogenic fibrosing alveolitis
   D   Empyema
   E   Asbestosis

32. **Uraemic pericarditis:**
   A   Commonly progresses to constrictive pericarditis
   B   Rarely produces tamponade
   C   Is often painless
   D   Usually occurs with low levels of blood urea
   E   Occurs only in chronic renal disease

33. **Causes of mononeuritis multiplex include:**
   A   Sarcoidosis
   B   Polyarteritis nodosa
   C   Diabetes mellitus
   D   Vitamin B deficiency
   E   Nitrofurantoin therapy

34. **Granulomatous uveitis is seen with:**
   A   Syphilis
   B   Diabetes mellitus
   C   Tuberculosis
   D   Ankylosing spondylitis
   E   Toxoplasmosis

35. **Diabetes mellitus may produce:**
   A   Monoarticular arthritis
   B   Charcot's-type joints
   C   Chondrocalcinosis
   D   Dupuytren's contractures
   E   Cutaneous calcification

36. **In the following, inheritance is sex-linked:**
   A   Alkaptonuria
   B   Duchenne's pseudohypertrophic muscular dystrophy
   C   Congenital non-endemic goitrous hypothyroidism
   D   Haemophilia A
   E   Hypophosphataemic rickets

37. **A red eye is found in:**
   A   Blepharitis
   B   Hypocalcaemia
   C   Conjunctivitis
   D   Chlorpropamide overdosage
   E   Iridocyclitis

38. **Dressler's syndrome is associated with:**
   A   Cardiac surgery
   B   Blunt trauma to the chest
   C   Pericardial effusion
   D   Horner's syndrome
   E   Recurrent attacks

39. **Male pattern body hair distribution in a female is seen in:**
    A   Myxoedema
    B   True hermaphroditism
    C   Laurence–Moon–Biedl syndrome
    D   Stein–Leventhal syndrome (polycystic ovarian disease)
    E   Cushing's syndrome

40. **Neuromuscular disturbances in chronic renal failure include:**
    A   Psychosis
    B   Flapping tremors
    C   Fasciculations commonly
    D   Peripheral neuropathy
    E   Bilateral lower motor neurone VIIth nerve palsy

41. **Incidence of carcinoma of the bronchus is increased with:**
    A   Exposure to beryllium
    B   Mining of radioactive ores
    C   Exposure to aflatoxins
    D   Manufacture of chromates
    E   Coal mining

42. **Hyponatraemia is associated with:**
    A   Hyperlipidaemia
    B   Adrenal cortical hyperfunction
    C   Inappropriate antidiuretic hormone secretion
    D   Hypoproteinaemia
    E   Dehydration

43. **Central cyanosis may be found in:**
    A   Methaemoglobinaemia
    B   Ventilation–perfusion defects
    C   Pulmonary arteriovenous fistula
    D   Heat stroke
    E   Severe exercise

44. **Jarisch–Herxheimer reactions are described with:**
   A Erythromycin therapy in Legionaire's disease
   B Penicillin therapy in syphilis
   C Tetracycline therapy in brucellosis
   D Dapsone therapy in leprosy
   E Steroid therapy in sarcoidosis

45. **Delirium may be produced by the following drugs:**
   A Barbiturates
   B Bromides
   C Salicylates in therapeutic doses
   D Hyoscine derivatives
   E Oral penicillin therapy

46. **The following statements characterize delirium tremens:**
   A Chlormethiazole (Heminevrin) is a useful drug
   B Auditory hallucinations occur
   C Visual hallucinations occur
   D Electroconvulsive therapy may be indicated in severe cases
   E The condition may be fatal

47. **The following statements are true about autism:**
   A It strongly suggests schizophrenia
   B Speech disorders occur
   C It predominantly occurs in children of obsessive-compulsive parents
   D Children may show obsessional disturbances
   E An organic basis is often demonstrable

48. **In Still's disease (Juvenile rheumatoid arthritis)**
   A Leukocytosis is usual
   B There is an association with HLA B27
   C Peak occurrence is at 12 years of age
   D Cervical spine involvement is rare
   E Prognosis is worse than in the adult form

49. **In brucellosis:**
   A   Splenomegaly is often tender
   B   Sterile pyuria is a feature
   C   Human-to-human transmission is common
   D   Calcification of the liver may be seen
   E   Chloramphenicol should be given for 2–3 weeks

50. **Varicella:**
   A   Causes a vesicular rash
   B   Is uncommon in adults
   C   Has an incubation period of 14–21 days
   D   Is infectious for one week following the rash
   E   Frequently develops herpes zoster after the initial infection

51. **Psittacosis is characterized by:**
   A   Leukocytosis
   B   Splenomegaly in the first week
   C   Macular rash
   D   Frank pulmonary consolidation on chest x-ray
   E   Common development of meningitis

52. **Renal failure is a common cause of death in:**
   A   Hypernephroma
   B   Systemic lupus erythematosus
   C   Weil's disease
   D   Renal tuberculosis
   E   Accelerated hypertension

53. **The following are curative with penicillin treatment in syphilis:**
   A   Meningitis
   B   Aortic aneurysm
   C   Interstitial keratitis
   D   Condyloma lata
   E   Generalized paresis of the insane

54. **Typical features of Mycoplasma pneumonia include:**
   A The common occurrence of pleural effusions
   B The very commonly seen presence of cold agglutinins
   C Associated renal failure
   D Good response to tetracyclines
   E Immunity in debilitated individuals if immunized against Mycoplasma

55. **Staphylococcal infections are commonly seen with:**
   A Diabetes mellitus
   B Mucoviscidosis
   C Chronic malaria
   D Tetracycline therapy
   E Variola infections

56. **Massive splenomegaly is characteristic of:**
   A Kala–azar
   B Iron–deficiency anaemia
   C Infectious mononucleosis
   D Myelofibrosis
   E Chronic myeloid leukaemia

57. **The following suggest a functional brain disorder:**
   A Auditory hallucinations
   B Perseveration
   C Early morning waking
   D Absent pupillary responses to light
   E Feelings of insects crawling over skin

58. **Post–traumatic epilepsy:**
   A Always follows within one month of head injury
   B Regularly shows abnormalities on computerized axial tomography of the brain
   C Requires surgical treatment in most cases
   D Responds poorly to standard anticonvulsant therapy
   E May show characteristic electroencephalographic changes

59. **The following are true regarding the lateral pop-liteal nerve:**
   A   It is formed by L4–5 nerve roots
   B   It is a terminal branch of the sciatic nerve
   C   It may be damaged as it winds around the neck of the fibula
   D   It may be affected in sarcoidosis
   E   It supplies sensation to the medial aspect of the foot

60. **The following statements are true:**
   A   Equal vertical distances on a logarithmic scale measure equal proportionate differences
   B   Logarithmic scales measure percentage changes in a variable
   C   The area of the bars of a histogram is inversely related to the total frequency
   D   A normal distribution curve is equally divided by a perpendicular drawn from the peak of the curve
   E   The measure of dispersion is used to decribe the variability of values in a distribution around their central value

61

SURNAME	INITIALS
JOSHI	P

CANDIDATE NUMBER

THOU. 0 1 2 3 4 5 6 7 8 9
HUND. 0 1 2 3 4 5 6 7 8 9
TENS 0 1 2 3 4 5 6 7 8 9
UNITS 0 1 2 3 4 5 6 7 8 9

4	7	5	6

PAGE No.
1
▯

T means TRUE F means FALSE D means DO NOT KNOW

1. 1A 1B 1C 1D 1E (T F D)
2. 2A 2B 2C 2D 2E (T F D)
3. 3A 3B 3C 3D 3E (T F D)
4. 4A 4B 4C 4D 4E (T F D)
5. 5A 5B 5C 5D 5E (T F D)
6. 6A 6B 6C 6D 6E (T F D)
7. 7A 7B 7C 7D 7E (T F D)
8. 8A 8B 8C 8D 8E (T F D)
9. 9A 9B 9C 9D 9E (T F D)
10. 10A 10B 10C 10D 10E (T F D)
11. 11A 11B 11C 11D 11E (T F D)
12. 12A 12B 12C 12D 12E (T F D)
13. 13A 13B 13C 13D 13E (T F D)
14. 14A 14B 14C 14D 14E (T F D)
15. 15A 15B 15C 15D 15E (T F D)
16. 16A 16B 16C 16D 16E (T F D)
17. 17A 17B 17C 17D 17E (T F D)
18. 18A 18B 18C 18D 18E (T F D)
19. 19A 19B 19C 19D 19E (T F D)
20. 20A 20B 20C 20D 20E (T F D)
21. 21A 21B 21C 21D 21E (T F D)
22. 22A 22B 22C 22D 22E (T F D)
23. 23A 23B 23D 23C 23E (T F D)
24. 24A 24B 24C 24D 24E (T F D)
25. 25A 25B 25C 25D 25E (T F D)
26. 26A 26B 26C 26D 26E (T F D)
27. 27A 27B 27C 27D 27E (T F D)
28. 28A 28B 28C 28D 28E (T F D)
29. 29A 29B 29C 29D 29E (T F D)
30. 30A 30B 30C 30D 30E (T F D)

62

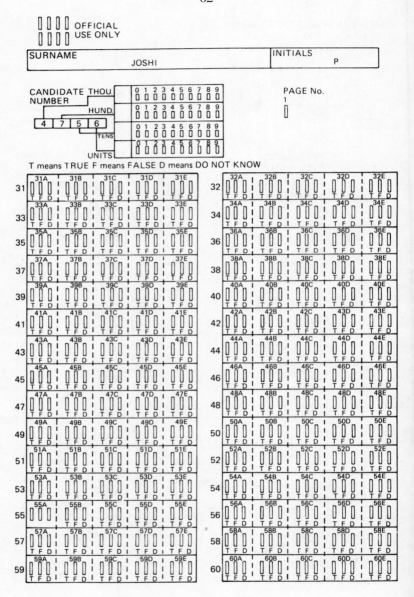

SURNAME   JOSHI   INITIALS   P

CANDIDATE THOU.   0 1 2 3 4 5 6 7 8 9   PAGE No.
NUMBER   1
                   HUND.   0 1 2 3 4 5 6 7 8 9
4 7 5 6
                   TENS   0 1 2 3 4 5 6 7 8 9

                   UNITS   0 1 2 3 4 5 6 7 8 9

T means TRUE F means FALSE D means DO NOT KNOW

Answers to Examination 3
(For complete References see Chapter 3)

1. A   False (erythema nodosum)
    B   True
    C   True
    D   True
    E   False
    Ref. (*3*) pp. 126, 199

2. A   False
    B   True
    C   False
    D   True
    E   True
    Ref. (*29*) pp. 118–119

3. A   False
    B   True
    C   True
    D   False (less than 10%)
    E   False
    Ref. (*8*) pp. 1088–1089, 1263–1264

4. A   True
    B   True
    C   True
    D   True
    E   True
    Ref. (*2*) pp. 1470–1472

5. A   True
    B   False
    C   True
    D   False
    E   True
    Ref. (*8*) pp. 1211, 1277–1278

6. A   True
    B   False
    C   True
    D   True
    E   False
    Ref. (*26*) pp. 378–382

7. A   True (dactylitis— common in children)
    B   True (adults)
    C   True
    D   False
    E   False
    Ref. (*2*) pp. 1547–1550

8. A   False
    B   False
    C   True
    D   True
    E   True
    Ref. (*3*) p. 139

9. A   False
    B   True
    C   False
    D   True
    E   True
    Ref. (*1*) pp. 71–82

10. A   False (large joints)
    B   True
    C   False
    D   False
    E   True
    Ref. (*2*) pp. 1885–1886

11. A True
     B False
     C True
     D False
     E True
     Ref. (*10*) pp. 498–504

12. A False
     B True
     C False
     D True
     E True
     Ref. (*6*) pp. 1275–1276

13. A False
     B True (if anaemia and leucopenia)
     C True (to prevent urate nephropathy)
     D False
     E True
     Ref. (*8*) pp. 1201–1202

14. A True
     B True
     C False (males)
     D False (tetracycline therapy)
     E False (poor)
     Ref. (*2*) pp. 757–759

15. A False (left atrium)
     B True
     C True
     D True
     E False (angiographic and echocardiographic changes)
     Ref. (*10*) p. 446

16. A False (autosomal dominant)
     B True
     C False
     D False (good response)
     E True
     Ref. (*8*) pp. 1210–1211

17. A True
     B True (because of coronary insufficiency)
     C False (normal)
     D False
     E True (one-third of cases)
     Ref. (*2*) pp. 1247–1249

18. A True
     B False
     C True
     D False
     E True (classical)
     Ref. (*27*) p. 282

19. A False
     B True
     C False
     D True
     E True
     Ref. (*28a*)

20. A True
     B False
     C True
     D False
     E True
     Ref. (*2*) pp. 1884–1885

21. A False
     B True (also colic,
        sweating and
        salivation)
     C True
     D False (meiosis—less
        than 3mm in size)
     E True
     Ref. (29)

22. A True
     B True
     C False (exudate)
     D True
     E True
     Ref. (30) p. 1319–1337

23. A False
        (non-deforming,
        large-joint
        involvement)
     B True (in 75%)
     C False
     D True (very
        common)
     E False (rare)
     Ref. (1) pp. 123–124

24. A False
     B False
     C True
     D True
     E True
     Ref. (2) p. 1134

25. A True
     B True
     C True
     D False
     E False
     Ref. (8) pp. 1214–1217

26. A False (partial)
     B False (constricted)
     C False (decreased)
     D False (IIIrd nerve
        palsy)
     E False
     Ref. (26) p. 32

27. A True
     B False
     C True
     D False
     E True
     Ref. (7) pp. 128–129

28. A True
     B True
     C True
     D False
        (hypoparathyroid-
        ism)
     E False (osteomalacia)
     Ref. (16)

29. A True
     B True
     C False
     D False
        (hypercalcaemia)
     E False
     Ref. (2) pp. 1503–1507

30. A True
     B False
     C True (temperature
        greater than 38°C)
     D False
     E True
     Ref. (2) pp. 1637–1639

31. A False
     B False
     C False
     D True
     E True
     Ref. (*9*) pp. 230, 250

32. A False
     B True
     C True
     D False
     E False
     Ref. (*2*) p. 1153

33. A True
     B True
     C True
     D False
     E False
     Ref. (*20*) p. 110

34. A True
     B False
     C True
     D False
        (non-
        granulomatous)
     E True
     Ref. (*23*) p. 112

35. A True (septic)
     B True
     C True
     D True
     E False
     Ref. (*1*) pp. 151–152

36. A False
     B True
     C False
     D True
     E True
     Ref. (*25*) pp. 1007–1008

37. A True
     B False
     C True
     D False
     E True
     Ref. (*23*) Inside of front
     cover

38. A False
        (postcardiotomy
        syndrome)
     B False
     C True
     D False
     E True
     Ref. (*10*) p. 464

39. A False
     B False
     C False
     D True
     E True
     Ref. (*16*) pp. 175–178

40. A True
     B True
     C False
     D True
     E False
     Ref. (*2*) pp. 1299–1307

41. A False
     B True
     C False
     D True
     E False
     Ref. (*8*) p. 895

42. A True
     B False
     C True
     D False
     E True
     Ref. (*5*) pp. 187–188

43. A   True
    B   True
    C   True
    D   False
    E   False
    Ref. (*9*) pp. 37–38

44. A   False
    B   True
    C   True
    D   True
    E   False
    Ref. (*2*) p. 725, (*8*)

45. A   True
    B   True
    C   False
    D   True
    E   False
    Ref. (*7*)

46. A   True
    B   True
    C   True
    D   False
    E   True
    Ref. (*2*) pp. 973–974

47. A   False (relationship
         controversial)
    B   True
    C   True
    D   True
    E   False
    Ref. (*2*) pp. 2012–2013

48. A   True about
         50 000/mm^3
    B   True
    C   False (1–3 years)
    D   False (frequent and
         early)
    E   False
    Ref. (*1*) pp. 65–70

49. A   True
    B   True
    C   False (very rare)
    D   True
    E   False (tetracyclines)
    Ref. (*2*) pp. 958–960

50. A   True
    B   False
    C   True
    D   False (for 24 hours
         before the rash)
    E   False
    Ref. (*2*) pp. 801–804

51. A   False (leucopenia)
    B   True
    C   True
    D   False
    E   False
    Ref. (*2*) pp. 769–771

52. A   False
    B   True
    C   True
    D   False
    E   True
    Ref. (*5*)

53. A   True
    B   False
    C   False
    D   True
    E   False
    Ref. (*2*) pp. 723–725

54. A   False
    B   True (90%)
    C   False
    D   True
    E   False (no vaccine is
         available)
    Ref. (*2*) pp. 760–761

55. A   True
    B   True
    C   False
    D   True
    E   False
    Ref. (*9*)

56. A   True
    B   False
    C   False
    D   True
    E   True
    Ref. (*20*) p. 37

57. A   True
    B   False (organic)
    C   True (endogenous
        depression)
    D   False
    E   True
    Ref. (*19*) pp. 119–159

58. A   False
    B   False
    C   False
    D   False
    E   True
    Ref. (*2*) p. 1948

59. A   False (L4, 5, S1, 2)
    B   True
    C   True
    D   True (mononeuritis
        multiplex)
    E   False
    Ref. (*14*) pp. 306–308

60. A   True
    B   True
    C   False (directly
        related)
    D   True
    E   True
    Ref. (*17*)

Examination 4

(Time allotted: 2½ hours)

1. **Miliary shadows on chest x-ray may be seen in:**
   A   Lymphangitis carcinomatosa
   B   Silicosis
   C   Tight mitral stenosis
   D   Severe pulmonary stenosis
   E   Alveolar proteinosis

2. **Raynaud's phenomenon is described with:**
   A   Myxoedema
   B   Ergot poisoning
   C   Severe hypothermia
   D   Cervical rib
   E   Systemic sclerosis

3. **Spider naevi characteristically occur with:**
   A   Chlorpromazine therapy
   B   Chronic vasodilator therapy
   C   Chronic active hepatitis
   D   Alcoholic cirrhosis
   E   Late pregnancy

4. **In a patient with macroglossia one would suspect:**
   A   Acromegaly
   B   Marfan's syndrome
   C   Hurler's syndrome
   D   Achondroplasia
   E   Amyloidosis

5. **Hyperkeratosis on the palms and soles is found in:**
   A   Hypovitaminosis A
   B   Arsenic poisoning
   C   Gonococcal septicaemia
   D   Tertiary syphilis
   E   Behçet's disease

6. **Paradoxical splitting of the 2nd heart sound is found in:**
   A   Severe pulmonary stenosis
   B   Ventricular septal defect
   C   Severe aortic stenosis
   D   Patent ductus arteriosus
   E   Complete right bundle-branch block

7. **Bilateral parotid enlargement is a feature of:**
   A   Mikulicz's syndrome
   B   Infectious mononucleosis
   C   Mumps
   D   Brucellosis
   E   Sarcoidosis

8. **Rib notching may be found with:**
   A   Patent ductus arteriosus
   B   Coarctation of the aorta
   C   Pulmonary arteriovenous fistula
   D   Neurofibromatosis
   E   Hypertrophic polyneuropathy

9. **Secondary hypertension is described with:**
   A   Fibromuscular hyperplasia of the renal artery
   B   Polycythaemia rubra vera
   C   Cushing's syndrome
   D   Zollinger–Ellison syndrome
   E   Antacid therapy

10. **In Conn's syndrome:**
    A   Serum aldosterone levels are characteristically raised
    B   Plasma renin activity is increased
    C   Hypertension is malignant in 10% of cases
    D   Hyperkalaemia is common
    E   Surgical therapy is of value

11. **Liver damage may be produced by:**
    A   Carbon tetrachloride
    B   Tetracyclines
    C   Cinchophen
    D   Muscarine aminata
    E   Chloroform

12. **Causes of nodular hepatomegaly include:**
    A   Postnecrotic cirrhosis
    B   Primary biliary cirrhosis
    C   Hepatic syphilis
    D   Weil's disease (Leptospira icterohaemorrhagia)
    E   Metastatic disease

13. **Giant 'a' waves are seen in:**
    A   Atrial fibrillation
    B   Nodal tachycardia
    C   Complete heart block
    D   Ventricular tachycardia
    E   Ventricular fibrillation

14. **Bronchiectasis is described in:**
    A   Measles bronchopneumonia
    B   Kartagener's syndrome
    C   Bronchial asthma
    D   Hepatic cirrhosis
    E   Scleroderma

15. **Turner's syndrome is associated with:**
    A   Infantilism
    B   Congenital abnormalities of the genitalia
    C   Atrial septal defect
    D   Retinitis pigmentosa
    E   Dwarfism

16. **Pulmonary fibrosis occurs with:**
    A   Dermatomyositis
    B   Nitrofurantoin therapy
    C   Morphoea
    D   Diabetes mellitus
    E   Cystic bronchiectasis

17. **Iritis is an associated feature of:**
    A   Whooping cough
    B   Rubella
    C   Syphilis
    D   Ankylosing spondylitis
    E   Toxoplasmosis

18. **The following are true regarding Endomyocardial fibrosis:**
    A   Young Africans are affected
    B   Clinical features resemble constrictive pericarditis
    C   A pansystolic murmur at the left sternal border which increases on inspiration is characteristic
    D   The treatment is surgical
    E   The electrocardiogram is diagnostic

19. **An arterial P_{CO_2} of 65mmHg is compatible with:**
    A   40% oxygen therapy in a patient with chronic obstructive pulmonary disease
    B   Ankylosing spondylitis
    C   Salicylate overdosage
    D   Barbiturate overdosage
    E   Pyloric stenosis

20. **The following features suggest an acute exacerbation of ulcerative colitis:**
    A   Development of anaemia
    B   Vertigo following sulphasalazine ingestion
    C   Macroscopic blood in the stool
    D   Development of a generalized rash
    E   Raised erythrocyte sedimentation rate

21. **With regards to the biliary system the following are true:**
   A The right and left hepatic ducts fuse to form the common bile duct
   B The common bile duct passes anterior to the duodenum to open in the duodenum
   C The gall bladder normally holds about 10 ml of bile
   D Gall-stones may become lodged in Hartmann's pouch
   E Gangrene of the gall bladder may be related to cystic artery thrombosis

. 22. **Toxic effects of imipramine include:**
   A Marked sweating
   B Obstructive jaundice
   C Photosensitization
   D Postural hypotension
   E Nephrogenic diabetes insipidus

23. **Early manifestations of congenital syphilis include:**
   A Eczema oris
   B Interstitial keratitis
   C Rubbery discrete occipital lymphadenopathy
   D Clutton's joints
   E Choroidoretinitis

24. **In congenital hypertrophic pyloric stenosis:**
   A The female is more frequently affected
   B There is an increased risk of affliction in the later offspring
   C The vomitus is almost never bile-stained
   D Barium meal is the investigation of choice and should be done early
   E Most patients require surgery

25. **Recognized indications for tonsillectomy include:**
   A Persistent visible enlargement of the cervical lymph nodes
   B Recurrent acute follicular tonsillitis
   C Sinobronchitis
   D Acute poliomyelitis
   E Congenital hypogammaglobulinaemia

26. **Haemophilia A:**
   A   Is inherited as a sex-linked recessive trait
   B   Commonly manifests during the first year of life
   C   Is excluded by absence of a family history of haemophilia
   D   Produces a prolonged bleeding time
   E   Produces a normal one-stage prothrombin time

27. **The following statements are true:**
   A   Up to 3000 ml urine/24 hours may be passed normally
   B   The amount of proteinuria indicates the severity of the renal lesion
   C   Granular casts are found only in renal disease
   D   Orthostatic proteinuria, if chronic, is harmful
   E   Tamm Horsfall protein is a normal constituent of urine

28. **Frank haematuria is consistent with:**
   A   Tuberculosis of the renal tract
   B   Acute pyelonephritis
   C   Acute cystitis
   D   Malignant hypertension
   E   Renal infarction

29. **The following statements apply to medullary sponge kidneys:**
   A   It is very uncommon
   B   It commonly presents in childhood
   C   The diagnosis is made radiologically
   D   The patient may present with renal stones
   E   Renal function is frequently impaired

30. **In acute intermittent porphyria:**
   A   Onset is usually in childhood
   B   Barbiturates are indicated if the patient is confused
   C   Peripheral neuropathy is common
   D   Sinus tachycardia is common during attacks
   E   Pethidine is contraindicated

31. **In Carcinoid syndrome:**
    A   The occurrence of mitral stenosis has been described
    B   Diagnosis is made by measuring vanillyl mandelic acid in the urine
    C   Methysergide has been used therapeutically
    D   Flushing attacks are often precipitated by alcohol
    E   Persistent wheezing is a recognized feature

32. **Primary optic atrophy is a recognized feature of:**
    A   Glaucoma
    B   Disseminated sclerosis
    C   Paget's disease of the skull
    D   Neurosyphilis
    E   Ethambutol therapy

33. **Typical features of Huntington's chorea include:**
    A   Autosomal dominant inheritance
    B   Progressive dementia
    C   Control of choreiform movements with tetrabenazine in some cases
    D   Optic atrophy
    E   Predominance in the male

34. **Predominantly, motor neuropathy is found in:**
    A   Diabetes mellitus
    B   Porphyria
    C   Guillain–Barré syndrome
    D   Friedrich's ataxia
    E   Diptheria

35. **Known causes of hypercholesterolaemia are:**
    A   Primary biliary cirrhosis
    B   Nephrotic syndrome
    C   Hyperthyroidism
    D   Hepatocellular jaundice
    E   Gaucher's disease

36. **Recognized causes of hepatic venous occlusion include:**
   A   Severe vomiting
   B   Senecio poisoning
   C   Hypernephroma
   D   Aflatoxin contamination
   E   Polycythaemia rubra vera

37. **A reduced glucose level in the pleural fluid with a normal blood sugar is recognized in:**
   A   Systemic lupus erythematosus
   B   Rheumatoid arthritis
   C   Severe pulmonary infarction
   D   Malignant effusion
   E   Tuberculosis

38. **The following are true regarding Charcot's joints:**
   A   Syringomyelia may be a cause
   B   Diabetes mellitus is a recognized cause
   C   It is commoner in women than in men
   D   Kyphosis may be a sequel
   E   If syphilitic in origin, penicillin therapy is curative

39. **The shoulder–hand syndrome is characterized by:**
   A   A painful and puffy swelling
   B   Frequently associated vasomotor changes
   C   An aetiological relationship to cervical osteoarthritis
   D   Pain being usually segmental in distribution
   E   Ankylosis and deformity

40. **In megaloblastic anaemia:**
   A   Serum vitamin B_{12} levels are always low
   B   Ascorbic acid deficiency may be causally related
   C   Confusion may be a presenting symptom
   D   Premature greying of the hair may be characteristic
   E   Jaundice is usually due to hepatocellular damage

41. **Syncopal attacks are well recognized in:**
   A Narcolepsy
   B Performance of a Valsalva manoeuvre
   C Children with pertussis infection
   D Shy–Drager syndrome
   E Stokes–Adams syndrome

42. **Alcohol ingestion may be associated with:**
   A Auditory hallucinations
   B Amnesic syndrome
   C Severe pruritis
   D Marchiafava–Bignami syndrome
   E Mononeuritis multiplex

43. **Drug-induced ototoxicity is produced by:**
   A Furosemide
   B Bromocriptine
   C Lithium carbonate
   D Streptomycin
   E Choloroquine

44. **The following are true regarding thyrotoxicosis:**
   A There is a strong correlation between the presence of long-acting thyroid stimulator (LATS) and anti-thyroglobulin antibodies
   B The association of LATS with pretibial myxoedema is well recognized
   C Carbimazole is ineffective in patients who do not have LATS antibody in their serum
   D Thyroid stimulating hormone increases following treatment in thyrotoxic patients
   E Exophthalmos does not occur in the absence of circulating LATS

45. **In pulmonary alveolar proteinosis:**
A   Marked interstitial lung disease is common
B   The cause is accumulation of surfactant
C   The presentation is in adolescents
D   The FEV_1/FVC ratio is raised above normal
E   Serum lactic dehydrogenase levels are used as a guide in monitoring treatment

46. **Iron deficiency anaemia may produce:**
A   Pearly white scleras
B   Hepatosplenomegaly
C   Glossidynia
D   Menorrhagia
E   Neurological abnormalities

47. **Lymphogranuloma venereum:**
A   Is caused by a Chlamydia organism
B   Is associated with a painful primary genital lesion
C   Produces painless inguinal lymphadenopathy
D   Is commonly associated with suppuration of the inguinal glands
E   May be associated with rectal strictures

48. **The following are true regarding vitamin B_6 (pyridoxine):**
A   Deficiency predisposes to Bell's palsy
B   The chemically active form is the coenzyme pyridoxal phosphate
C   Deficiency in infants produces convulsions
D   Deficiency associated with isoniazid therapy may be related to the acetylator status of the patient
E   If high doses are used, rifampicin is inactivated

49. **In sickle–cell anaemia:**
A   Typhoid fever commonly occurs
B   An impaired ability to concentrate urine results
C   Clinical manifestations develop as the proportion of haemoglobin S (HbS) in the red cells increases
D   The anaemia is usually mild
E   Thrombocytopenia commonly results

50. **The following statements regarding hallucinations are true:**
   A Auditory hallucinations are common in amphetamine psychosis
   B Cocaine psychosis is characterized by paranoid changes
   C Slimming tablets may produce hallucinations
   D They are invariable in schizophrenia
   E Pure visual hallucinations are likely to indicate functional disease

51. **In encephalitis lethargica:**
   A Choreiform and athetoid movements are seen in the acute phase
   B Oculogyric crisis is seen following therapy
   C Endogenous depression is a frequently associated finding
   D Mental subnormality may be associated
   E Argyll Robertson pupils may be seen

52. **Psychosomatic disorders may be related to:**
   A Systemic lupus erythematosus
   B Vasomotor rhinitis
   C Peptic ulcers
   D Diabetes mellitus
   E Barter's syndrome

53. **The following antidotes are well recognized:**
   A Naloxone hydrochloride in morphine overdosage
   B Pralidoxime chloride in parathion poisoning
   C Dimercaprol in cyanide poisoning
   D Orphenadrine in pyridostigmine poisoning
   E Cobalt edetate in haloperidol overdosage

54. **HLA B8-associated diseases include:**
   A Multiple sclerosis
   B Dermatitis herpetiformis
   C Coeliac disease
   D Ankylosing spondylitis
   E Myasthenia gravis

55. **Aetiological factors in chronic pancreatitis are:**
   A   Alcohol
   B   Primary hyperparathyroidism
   C   Thiazide diuretic therapy
   D   Corticosteroid therapy
   E   Type III hyperlipoproteinaemia

56. **Primary hyperparathyroidism may present with:**
   A   Looser's zones on x-ray
   B   Psychosis
   C   Constipation
   D   Brachymetacarpal dwarfism
   E   Nephrocalcinosis

57. **Herpes simplex encephalitis:**
   A   Produces an acute necrotizing encephalitis
   B   Neutralizing antibody titres may help in the diagnosis
   C   It is often localized to one part of the brain
   D   Gentian violet 1% is used systemically as therapy
   E   Brain biopsy may be required to make a diagnosis

58. **Brucellosis commonly presents with:**
   A   Bilateral hilar lymphadenopathy on chest x-ray
   B   Jaundice
   C   Illness for weeks to months with spontaneous remissions
   D   Splenomegaly
   E   Pronounced sweating

59. **The following statements are true regarding anthrax:**
   A   It is an occupational disease
   B   Woolsorters' disease is produced by inhalation
   C   Over 90% of patients present with skin involvement
   D   The malignant pustule is severely painful
   E   Regional lymphadenopathy is very unusual

60. **The following statements are true:**
    A Equal distances on an arithmetic scale measure equal absolute differences
    B Curves of frequency distribution always assume the same shape
    C The arithmetic mean is the 'average' of a collection of values
    D The median divides the observations in two equal groups when arranged in an ascending order of magnitude
    E The median is always equal to the arithmetic mean

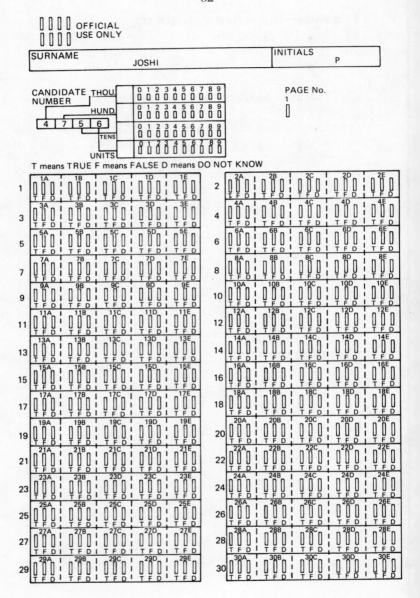

82

OFFICIAL USE ONLY

SURNAME JOSHI

INITIALS P

CANDIDATE NUMBER

4 7 5 6

PAGE No.
1

T means TRUE F means FALSE D means DO NOT KNOW

83

 OFFICIAL
USE ONLY

SURNAME	INITIALS
JOSHI	P

CANDIDATE THOU.
NUMBER

| 0 1 2 3 4 5 6 7 8 9 | | | | | | | | | |

HUND.

| 0 1 2 3 4 5 6 7 8 9 | | | | | | | | | |

| 4 | 7 | 5 | 6 |

TENS

| 0 1 2 3 4 5 6 7 8 9 | | | | | | | | | |

UNITS

| 0 1 2 3 4 5 6 7 8 9 | | | | | | | | | |

PAGE No.
1

T means TRUE F means FALSE D means DO NOT KNOW

	31A	31B	31C	31D	31E		32A	32B	32C	32D	32E
31	T F D	T F D	T F D	T F D	T F D	32	T F D	T F D	T F D	T F D	T F D
33	33A	33B	33C	33D	33E	34	34A	34B	34C	34D	34E
	T F D	T F D	T F D	T F D	T F D		T F D	T F D	T F D	T F D	T F D
35	35A	35B	35C	35D	35E	36	36A	36B	36C	36D	36E
	T F D	T F D	T F D	T F D	T F D		T F D	T F D	T F D	T F D	T F D
37	37A	37B	37C	37D	37E	38	38A	38B	38C	38D	38E
	T F D	T F D	T F D	T F D	T F D		T F D	T F D	T F D	T F D	T F D
39	39A	39B	39C	39D	39E	40	40A	40B	40C	40D	40E
	T F D	T F D	T F D	T F D	T F D		T F D	T F D	T F D	T F D	T F D
41	41A	41B	41C	41D	41E	42	42A	42B	42C	43D	43E
	T F D	T F D	T F D	T F D	T F D		T F D	T F D	T F D	T F D	T F D
43	43A	43B	43C	43D	43E	44	44A	44B	44C	44D	44E
	T F D	T F D	T F D	T F D	T F D		T F D	T F D	T F D	T F D	T F D
45	45A	45B	45C	45D	45E	46	46A	46B	46C	46D	46E
	T F D	T F D	T F D	T F D	T F D		T F D	T F D	T F D	T F D	T F D
47	47A	47B	47C	47D	47E	48	48A	48B	48C	48D	48E
	T F D	T F D	T F D	T F D	T F D		T F D	T F D	T F D	T F D	T F D
49	49A	49B	49C	49D	49E	50	50A	50B	50C	50D	50E
	T F D	T F D	T F D	T F D	T F D		T F D	T F D	T F D	T F D	T F D
51	51A	51B	51C	51D	51E	52	52A	52B	52C	52D	52E
	T F D	T F D	T F D	T F D	T F D		T F D	T F D	T F D	T F D	T F D
53	53A	53B	53C	53D	53E	54	54A	54B	54C	54D	54E
	T F D	T F D	T F D	T F D	T F D		T F D	T F D	T F D	T F D	T F D
55	55A	55B	55C	55D	55E	56	56A	56B	56C	56D	56E
	T F D	T F D	T F D	T F D	T F D		T F D	T F D	T F D	T F D	T F D
57	57A	57B	57C	57D	57E	58	58A	58B	58C	58D	58E
	T F D	T F D	T F D	T F D	T F D		T F D	T F D	T F D	T F D	T F D
59	59A	59B	59C	59D	59E	60	60A	60B	60C	60D	60E
	T F D	T F D	T F D	T F D	T F D		T F D	T F D	T F D	T F D	T F D

Answers to Examination 4
(For complete References see Chapter 3)

1. A True
   B True
   C True
   D False
   E False
   Ref. (9) pp. 51, 205, 206

2. A False
   B True
   C False
   D True
   E True
   Ref. (24) pp. 68, 104, 109,
   130, 138, 152, 247, 267

3. A False
   B False
   C True
   D True
   E True
   Ref. (24) p. 270
       (20) pp. 31, 32, 35, 39,
   200

4. A True
   B False
   C True
   D False
   E True
   Ref. (22) pp. 77, 444

5. A True
   B True
   C False
   D False
   E False
   Ref. (3) p. 225

6. A False
   B False
   C True
   D True
   E False (left
       bundle-branch
       block)
   Ref. (2) p. 996

7. A True
   B False
   C True (painful)
   D False
   E True
   Ref. (24) p. 67

8. A False
   B True
   C False
   D True
   E True
   Ref. (24) p. 241

9. A True
   B True (rarely)
   C True
   D False
   E False
   Ref. (24) p. 252

10. A True
    B False
    C False (almost always
        benign)
    D False (hypokalaemia)
    E True
    Ref. (16) p. 38

11. A True
     B True
     C True
     D True
     E True
     Ref. (*20*) p. 196

12. A True
     B False
     C True
     D False
     E True
     Ref. (*24*) pp. 269–270

13. A False
     B True
     C True
     D True
     E False
     Ref. (*24*) p. 206

14. A True (also whooping cough)
     B True (with associated dextrocardia, frontal sinus aplasia)
     C False
     D False
     E False
     Ref. (*9*) pp. 114–121

15. A True
     B True
     C False (coarctation of the aorta)
     D False (red–green blindness)
     E True
     Ref. (*16*) p. 79

16. A True
     B True
     C False (localized scleroderma)
     D False
     E True
     Ref. (*9*) p. 237

17. A False
     B False
     C True
     D True
     E True
     Ref. (*20*) p. 24

18. A True
     B True
     C True (tricuspid incompetence)
     D False
     E False
     Ref. (*10*) p. 443

19. A True (because of removal of the hypoxic drive to respiration)
     B True
     C False (respiratory alkalosis and metabolic acidosis)
     D True (secondary to respiratory depression)
     E False
     Ref. (*9*)

20. A True
     B False
     C True
     D False
     E True
     Ref. (*18*) p. 178

21. A   False (common
         hepatic duct)
     B   False (posteriorly)
     C   False (50 cc)
     D   True
     E   True (extremely
         rare)
     Ref. (*14*) pp. 117–121

22. A   True
     B   True (allergic type)
     C   True (similar to
         phenothiazines)
     D   True
     E   False (lithium
         carbonate)
     Ref. (*7*) p. 263

23. A   True (due to
         associated nasal
         osteitis)
     B   False (sudden onset
         at about 6–8 years)
     C   True (very
         common)
     D   False (late
         manifestation)
     E   False (late
         manifestation)
     Ref. (*2*) pp. 720–721, 723,
     724

24. A   False (M:F :: 4:1)
     B   False (usually 1st
         born)
     C   True
     D   False
     E   False (most patients
         respond to
         Eumydrin)
     Ref. (*15*) p. 321

25. A   True
     B   True
     C   False
     D   False
     E   False
     Ref. (*31*) p. 154

26. A   True
     B   False
     C   False (fairly high
         mutation rate)
     D   False (increased
         clotting time)
     E   True
     Ref. (*55*) p. 516

27. A   True
     B   False
     C   True
     D   False
     E   True
     Ref. (*55*) pp. 383–385

28. A   True
     B   False
     C   True
     D   False
     E   True
     Ref. (*55*) p. 385

29. A   False (not
         uncommon)
     B   False (the age of
         onset is from
         childhood to late
         adulthood,
         presenting most
         commonly between
         the 4th and 7th
         decades of life)
     C   True
     D   True
     E   False (unless
         secondary to infection
         or stones)
     Ref. (*55*) pp. 411–412

30. A False
    B False (it may
       precipitate an attack)
    C True
    D True
    E False
    Ref. (55) p. 463

31. A True (if it is due to a
       bronchial adenoma)
    B False (5-hydroxy-
       indoleacetic acid)
    C True (it blocks the
       action of 5-hydroxy-
       tryptamine)
    D True
    E True
    Ref. (2) pp. 476–479

32. A False (consecutive
       optic atrophy)
    B True
    C False
    D True
    E True
    Ref. (24) p. 300

33. A True
    B True
    C True
    D False
    E False (sexes are
       equally affected)
    Ref. (26) pp. 288–299

34. A False
       (predominantly
       sensory)
    B True
    C True
    D False
    E True
    Ref. (2) pp. 2029–2035

35. A True
    B True
    C False (myxoedema)
    D False (obstructive
       jaundice)
    E False
    Ref. (2) pp. 1161–1163

36. A False
    B True
    C True (by producing
       occlusion of the
       inferior vena cava)
    D False (related to
       hepatoma)
    E True (most often the
       cause)
    Ref. (2) pp. 1479, 1480

37. A False
    B True
    C False
    D True
    E True
    Ref. (30) pp. 1346–1347

38. A True (classically in
       upper extremities)
    B True
    C False (commoner in
       men)
    D True
    E False (no satisfactory
       medical treatment)
    Ref. (1) pp. 151–152

39. A True
    B True
    C True
    D False
    E False
    Ref. (2) p. 1903

40. A   False (may be folate deficiency)
    B   False (produces macrocytic anaemia)
    C   True
    D   True (Addisonian pernicious anaemia)
    E   False (haemolytic jaundice)
    Ref. (2) pp. 1518–1525

41. A   False
    B   True
    C   True (following bouts of coughing)
    D   True (degeneration of lateral horn cells and basal ganglia)
    E   True
    Ref. (26) pp. 172–175
        (8) p. 1355

42. A   True (in delirium tremens)
    B   True (Korsakoff's psychosis)
    C   False
    D   True (callosal demyelinating encephalopathy)
    E   False
    Ref. (2) pp. 971–975

43. A   True (also ethycrinic acid)
    B   False
    C   False
    D   True
    E   True
    Ref. (6)

44. A   True
    B   True
    C   False
    D   True
    E   False
    Ref. (33) pp. 176–177

45. A   False
    B   True
    C   False
    D   True
    E   True
    Ref. (30) pp. 1253–1256

46. A   True
    B   True
    C   True
    D   False
    E   False
    Ref. (2) pp. 1514–1517

47. A   True
    B   False (painless)
    C   False
    D   True
    E   True
    Ref. (2) pp. 767–769

48. A   False
    B   True
    C   True
    D   True
    E   False
    Ref. (2) pp. 427–428

49. A   False
    B   True
    C   True
    D   False
    E   False
    Ref. (2) pp. 1547–1550

50. A   True
     B   True
     C   True
     D   False
     E   False (indicate
          organic disease)
     Ref. (28b) p. 269

51. A   True
     B   False
     C   False (reactive)
     D   True
     E   False
     Ref. (35) p. 151

52. A   False
     B   True
     C   True
     D   True
     E   False
     Ref. (35) p. 120

53. A   True
     B   True
     C   False
     D   False
     E   False
     Ref. (28b) p. 206

54. A   False (A3, B7,
          D2, B group 4)
     B   True
     C   True
     D   False (HLA B27)
     E   True
     Ref. (28c) pp. 449–458

55. A   True
     B   True
     C   False
     D   False
     E   False (types I, IV and
          V)
     Ref. (28d) p. 553

56. A   False (osteomalacia)
     B   True
     C   True
     D   False (pseudo-
          pseudohypo-
          parathyroidism)
     E   True
     Ref. (2) pp. 1832–1839

57. A   True
     B   True
     C   True
     D   False
     E   True
     Ref. (2) pp. 848–849

58. A   False
     B   False
     C   True
     D   True
     E   True
     Ref. (2) pp. 658–660

59. A   True
     B   True
     C   True
     D   False
     E   False
     Ref. (2) pp. 667–668

60. A   True
     B   False (may assume
          any particular shape)
     C   True
     D   True
     E   False
     Ref. (17)

Examination 5

(Time allotted: 2½ hours)

1. **Nephroblastoma (Wilm's tumour):**
   A   Is a malignant tumour of childhood
   B   Develops distant spread rapidly
   C   May present with systemic hypertension
   D   If localized, nephrectomy is indicated
   E   May produce hypercalcaemia

2. **Pleural fluid glucose of less than 60 mg% (3.3 mmol/litre) in the presence of a normal blood sugar is found in:**
   A   Acute pancreatitis
   B   Severe congestive cardiac failure
   C   Meig's syndrome
   D   Parapneumonic effusion
   E   Rheumatoid arthritis

3. **Recognized causes of nephrotic syndrome include:**
   A   Constrictive pericarditis
   B   Malaria
   C   Goodpasture's syndrome
   D   Hodgkin's disease
   E   Excessive ingestion of phenacetin

4. **Acute rheumatic fever may be associated with the following electrocardiographic changes:**
   A Shortened Q–T interval
   B Non-paroxysmal atrioventricular nodal tachycardia
   C Prominent 'u' waves
   D Second degree atrioventricular block
   E Delta waves

5. **Clinical manifestations of Leriche's syndrome include:**
   A Loss of libido
   B Sciatica
   C Symmetric atrophy of the legs
   D Absence of femoral pulses
   E Dilated collaterals over the thorax

6. **Secondary hypogammaglobulinaemia may be found with:**
   A Dystrophia myotonica
   B Thoracic duct fistula
   C Paroxysmal nocturnal haemoglobinaemia
   D Diazoxide therapy
   E Giant follicular lymphoma

7. **Subacute combined degeneration of the cord:**
   A May be associated with optic atrophy
   B Usually presents with numbness and paraesthesiae in the feet
   C Shows brisk abdominal reflexes
   D Produces motor abnormalities which resolve more completely than sensory ones
   E Commonly presents with a spastic paraparesis

8. **Non-cardiogenic pulmonary oedema is found with:**
   A Paracetamol overdosage
   B Nitrofurantoin therapy
   C Oxygen toxicity
   D Head injury
   E Ketoacidosis

9. **Hypoglycaemia is a feature of:**
   A   Addison's disease
   B   Zollinger–Ellison syndrome
   C   Chlorpropamide therapy
   D   High dose penicillin therapy
   E   Chlorpromazine therapy

10. **Crohn's disease—the following are correct:**
   A   Relatives of patients have a lower incidence of ulcerative colitis
   B   May present as a pyrexia of unknown aetiology
   C   Ankylosing spondylitis may precede gut manifestations
   D   Shows an increased risk of bowel carcinoma after 10 years
   E   Presenting diarrhoea is usually bloodless

11. **Neuropsychiatric disturbances of liver failure include:**
   A   Reversal of sleep pattern
   B   Argyll Robertson pupils
   C   Myelopathy with paraplegia
   D   Perseveration
   E   Diagnostic electroencephalographic changes

12. **Recognized features of rheumatoid arthritis include:**
   A   Posterior subcapsular cataracts
   B   Hoarseness
   C   Pancytopenia
   D   Renal amyloidosis
   E   Rapid response to low dose steroids

13. **Psoriatic arthritis:**
   A   Occurs in about 20% of psoriatics
   B   Joint involvment is usually symmetrical
   C   Sacroiliitis is characteristic
   D   Often shows minimal destructive changes in the joints of the hands
   E   Steroids are usually contraindicated

14. **With regards to x-ray skull features of raised intracranial pressure:**
   A   Suture diastasis is the most important finding in children
   B   Increased convolutional markings is a very reliable sign
   C   In the child, changes in the sella, are seen late
   D   Calcified pineal displacement is significant if shifted more than 3 mm
   E   In adults porosis is an unreliable finding

15. **Cranial nerve palsies in diabetes mellitus:**
   A   Are related to the severity of the disease
   B   Usually persist permanently
   C   If the pupil is dilated with a 3rd nerve lesion, posterior communicating artery aneurysm is a less likely diagnosis
   D   No treatment is required other than control of the diabetes
   E   6th nerve is the most frequently affected nerve

16. **Molluscum contagiosum:**
   A   Is a DNA virus of the pox family
   B   Is found only in humans
   C   Produces severely pruritic lesions
   D   Paracentric umbilication of the papules is characteristic
   E   Cantharadin application is effective therapy

17. **Mediastinal emphysema is manifested by:**
   A   Prominent suprasternal pulsations
   B   Hamman's sign (systolic crunch)
   C   Sore throat
   D   Gas under the diaphragm
   E   Cyanosis

18. **Transient loss of memory is recognized:**
   A   Following head injury
   B   In epileptics
   C   In vascular insufficiency
   D   In Alzheimer's disease
   E   In temporal lobe tumours

19. **Tingling paraesthesiae are typical of:**
   A   Multiple sclerosis
   B   Temporal lobe epilepsy
   C   Raynaud's phenomenon
   D   Acromegaly
   E   Hypoventilation

20. **Complications of non-gonococcal urethritis include:**
   A   Cataracts in newborns of infected mothers
   B   Urethral strictures
   C   Epididymitis
   D   Inclusion blenorrhoea
   E   Endocarditis

21. **Acute lactic acidosis:**
   A   Is suspected if the anion gap is greater than 15 mmol
   B   Is found in uraemia
   C   Is commonly associated with chlorpropamide therapy
   D   Usually produces a very low serum bicarbonate
   E   Should be treated with a lactate infusion

22. **In supravalvar aortic stenosis:**
   A   An early diastolic murmur is commonly heard
   B   An ejection click is characteristic
   C   Aortic dilatation is constant
   D   The physical appearance is often characteristic
   E   Peripheral pulmonary artery stenosis may coexist

23. **Elevated non-pulsating jugular veins may be seen with:**
   A   Superior mediastinal syndrome
   B   Massive pleural effusion
   C   Superior vena caval thrombosis
   D   Constrictive pericarditis
   E   Descending aortic aneurysm

24. **Cushing's syndrome is strongly suggested by:**
    A Cataracts
    B Hyperpigmentation
    C Diabetes mellitus
    D Extreme weakness and muscle wasting
    E Ecchymoses in the absence of thrombocytopenia

25. **Long-term corticosteroid therapy may be associated with:**
    A Hypochloraemic alkalosis
    B Positive nitrogen balance
    C Thrombophlebitis
    D Increased gastric acidity
    E Sleeplessness

26. **Hormones antagonizing insulin action include:**
    A Prolactin
    B Oestrogens
    C Adrenocorticotropic hormones
    D Thyroxin
    E Somatotropin

27. **Increased bone density is a feature of:**
    A Cushing's syndrome
    B Post-irradiation
    C Fluorosis
    D Vitamin A intoxication
    E Marble bone disease (osteopetrosis)

28. **Laurence – Moon – Biedl syndrome is characterized by:**
    A Peripheral neuropathy
    B Obesity
    C Retinitis pigmentosa
    D Hyperlipaemia
    E Mental retardation

29. **In coarctation of the aorta:**
   A   Congestive failure is usually secondary to hypertension
   B   Rupture of the aorta is a recognized association
   C   Cerebrovascular haemorrhage is a known hazard
   D   Infective endocarditis on the bicuspid valves is a frequent event
   E   Systolic hypertension without diastolic hypertension is most frequently present

30. **Cardiac disease associated with a marked eosinophilia may be produced by:**
   A   Polyarteritis nodosa
   B   Eosinophilic leukaemia
   C   Trichinosis
   D   Endomyocardial fibrosis
   E   Visceral larva migrans

31. **The following statements regarding gout are true:**
   A   Hyperuricaemia is a prerequisite for the diagnosis
   B   Only the outer portion of a large tophus undergoes rapid exchange with the miscible pool
   C   Uric acid excretion occurs only through the kidneys
   D   Podagra ultimately occurs in about 90% of the cases
   E   Phagocytosis of urate crystals by polymorphonuclear leucocytes results in the pain produced in gout

32. **Pancreatic enzyme deficiency is well recognized in:**
   A   Chronic pancreatitis
   B   Pancreatic carcinoma
   C   Benign pancreatic cystadenoma
   D   Crohn's disease
   E   Zollinger–Ellison syndrome

33. **Recognized causes of clubbing include:**
   A   Fibrosing alveolitis
   B   Chronic obstructive airways disease
   C   Asbestosis, uncomplicated by malignancy
   D   Meig's syndrome
   E   Crohn's disease

34. **The following anatomical considerations are true:**
   A   Optic chiasma lesions characteristically produce a bitemporal hemianopia
   B   Central scotoma occurs early in papilloedema
   C   In cortical blindness pupillary reactions are abnormal
   D   Optic tract lesions produce an ipsilateral homonymous hemianopia
   E   Opticokinetic nystagmus is found with bilateral infarction of the parieto-occipital lobes

35. **Dementia may be caused by:**
   A   Pick's disease
   B   A meningioma
   C   Parkinson's disease
   D   Low pressure hydrocephalus
   E   Motor neurone disease

36. **Depression is recognized under the following circumstances:**
   A   Associated with chronic painful diseases
   B   Following glandular fever
   C   Associated with alphamethyldopa therapy
   D   Associated with chlorpromazine therapy
   E   In Alzheimer's disease

37. **Splenomegaly is found with:**
   A   Macroglobulinaemia
   B   Megaloblastic anaemia
   C   Hand–Schüller–Christian disease
   D   Constrictive pericarditis
   E   Hyperchylomicronaemia

38. **Rapid reduction of elevated blood pressure is effected by:**
   A   Intravenous propranolol
   B   Oral diazoxide
   C   Intramuscular hydrallazine
   D   Intravenous methyldopa
   E   Intravenous clonidine

39. **X-linked recessive inheritance is recognized in:**
   A   Tay–Sachs disease
   B   Diaphyseal achlasia
   C   Red–Green colour blindness
   D   Christmas disease (factor IX deficiency)
   E   Hunter's syndrome (mucopolysaccharidosis II)

40. **The following side-effects of drugs are described in the fetus:**
   A   Alcoholism producing microcephaly
   B   Sulphonylureas producing neural tube defects
   C   Chloroquine producing corneal opacities
   D   Cortisone producing cleft palates
   E   Tetracycline producing phocomelia

41. **A raised amniotic fluid alpha-fetoprotein level may indicate:**
   A   A neural tube defect
   B   Inheritable haemoglobinopathies
   C   Congenital nephrosis
   D   Turner's syndrome
   E   Cystic fibrosis (mucoviscidosis)

42. **The following statements regarding retinoblast-oma are true:**
   A   It is usually fatal even if diagnosis is made early
   B   Transmission is autosomal recessive
   C   They may occur bilaterally
   D   The finding of leukocorea suggests the diagnosis
   E   It may present with heterochromia

43. **A 36-year-old businessman is found to have a urinary output of 300 ml/24 hours and a blood urea of 25 mmol/litre (150 mg/100 ml). The possible causes include:**
   A   A connective tissue disorder
   B   Lithium carbonate therapy
   C   Dissection of the aorta
   D   Ethambutol toxicity
   E   Cephaloridine therapy

44. **Nephrotoxicity is described with the following drugs:**
    A   Gentamicin
    B   Polymixin B
    C   Acetazolamide
    D   Ampicillin
    E   Rifampicin

45. **Typical symptoms of the hyperventilation syndrome are:**
    A   Headaches worst on waking
    B   Visual disturbances
    C   Difficulty with walking in the dark
    D   Circumoral paraesthesiae
    E   Intention tremor

46. **Complications of blood transfusions include:**
    A   Fat embolism
    B   Haemolytic reactions
    C   Haemosiderosis
    D   Thrombocytopenia
    E   Hypercalcaemia

47. **The following diseases may inadvertently be transmitted by blood transfusions:**
    A   Cytomegalovirus infection
    B   Toxoplasmosis
    C   Herpes zoster
    D   *Dracunculus medinensis*
    E   Trypanosomiasis (Chagas's disease)

48. **Acute upper gastrointestinal bleeding is described in:**
    A   Pseudoxanthoma elasticum
    B   Ménétrièr's disease
    C   Hereditary telengiectasia
    D   Oesophagitis
    E   Excessive smoking

49. **The differential diagnosis of acute appendicitis includes:**
   A   Mesenteric adenitis
   B   Acute cholecystitis
   C   Perforated peptic ulcer
   D   Right basal pneumonia
   E   Torsion of an ovarian cyst

50. **Features strongly associated with oat-cell carcinoma of the lung are:**
   A   Inappropriate antidiuretic hormone production
   B   Hypercalcaemia
   C   Predominance in the female sex
   D   Development of carcinoma in pre-existing lung 'scars'
   E   Bronchorrhoea

51. **Hypothermia in the elderly:**
   A   Is usually due to an endocrine cause
   B   May be due to chlorpromazine therapy
   C   Should be treated by rapid rewarming
   D   May present with prolongation of muscular relaxation time
   E   May be related to thiamine deficiency

52. **In onchocerciasis:**
   A   Transmission is by the Simulium fly
   B   The living microfilariae provoke a marked inflammatory response
   C   Eye involvement is more likely when the nodules occur around the head
   D   Choroidoretinitis may be found
   E   Eye involvement should be rapidly treated with suramin

53. **Herpes simplex virus:**
   A   Is present in buccal mucosal cells of over 60% of adults
   B   Initial infection is usually severe
   C   Recurrent attacks of herpes labialis occur throughout life in those with absence of antibodies
   D   Commonly produces a vulvovaginitis
   E   Treatment is only symptomatic

54. **In Brucellosis:**
   A   *Brucella suis* is the commonest infecting organism in Britain
   B   Hepatic granulomata resembling tuberculosis may occur
   C   An undulant course is the commonest pattern in Britain
   D   Epistaxis is a very frequent presenting feature
   E   High dose penicillin is effective therapy

55. **Recognized complications of chronic renal failure include:**
   A   Severe motor-sensory peripheral neuropathy
   B   Metastatic calcification
   C   Hypercalcaemia
   D   Acute arthritis resembling gout
   E   Proximal myopathy

56. **In the serum sickness reaction:**
   A   Symptoms occur 6 weeks after an injection of horse serum
   B   Proteinuria is usually present
   C   The disease results from formation of antibody-antigen complexes
   D   Leucopenia is a common accompaniment
   E   Only steroids in high doses are of any value

57. **Side-effects of benzothiadiazides may include:**
   A   Hypercalcaemia
   B   Acute pancreatitis
   C   Hyperglycaemia
   D   Cholestatic jaundice
   E   Necrotizing vasculitis

58. **Nifedipine:**
   A   Is a benzodiazepine derivative
   B   May be used effectively in patients with Prinzmetal's angina
   C   Acts by inhibiting phosphodiesterase
   D   Is a potent coronary vasodilator
   E   Is contraindicated in myocardial infarction

59. **Circulating anticoagulants have been described in:**
   A   Rocky Mountain spotted fever
   B   Werlhof's disease
   C   Dysproteinaemias
   D   Systemic lupus erythematosus
   E   Haemophilia

60. **The following statements are true:**
   A   The mode is the most commonly occurring value
   B   The mode is usually different in value from the mean
   C   In distributions which are markedly skewed, the arithmetic mean is a more appropriate measure than the geometric mean
   D   The standard deviation is also referred to as the root mean square deviation
   E   In a positively skewed distribution, the mean always lies to the left of the mode

103

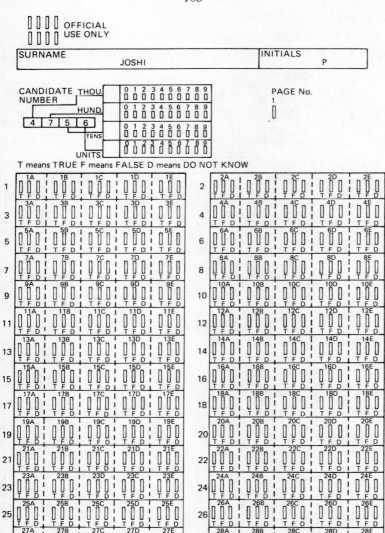

104

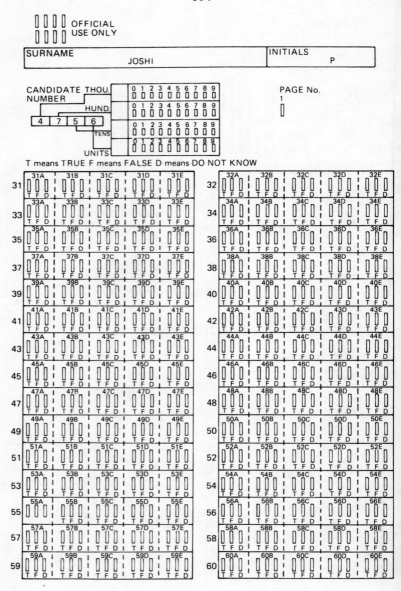

OFFICIAL USE ONLY

SURNAME JOSHI

INITIALS P

CANDIDATE NUMBER 4 7 5 6

PAGE No. 1

T means TRUE F means FALSE D means DO NOT KNOW

Answers to Examination 5
(For complete References see Chapter 3)

1. A True
   B True
   C True
   D True
   E False (seen with hypernephroma)
   Ref. (2) p. 1356

2. A False
   B False
   C False
   D True
   E True
   Ref. (30) pp. 1346–1347

3. A True
   B True
   C False
   D True
   E False
   Ref. (5) p. 67

4. A False (prolonged)
   B True
   C False
   D True
   E False
   Ref. (11) p. 298

5. A False
   B False
   C True
   D True
   E False
   Ref. (2) pp. 1181, 1183

6. A True
   B True
   C True
   D True
   E True
   Ref. (33) p. 84

7. A True
   B True
   C False (absent)
   D False
   E False (less commonly)
   Ref. (20) pp. 115–116

8. A False
   B False
   C True
   D True
   E True
   Ref. (30) p. 1320

9. A True
   B False
   C True
   D False
   E False
   Ref. (2) pp. 1758–1762

10. A False
    B True
    C True
    D False
    E True
    Ref. (2) pp. 1411–1416

11. A True
    B False
    C True
    D True
    E False
    Ref. (*41*) p. 135

12. A False (side-effects of
       steroids)
    B True (due to
       crico-arytenoid joint
       involvement)
    C True (Felty's
       syndrome—seen in
       5%)
    D True (20% on
       microscopy)
    E False
    Ref. (*2*) pp. 1872–1880

13. A True
    B False (asymmetrical)
    C True
    D False (highly
       destructive)
    E False (triamcinolone
       is most effective)
    Ref. (*2*) pp. 1884–1885

14. A True
    B False
    C True
    D True
    E False
    Ref. (*44*) pp. 1163–1166

15. A False
    B False (improves
       within 1–3 months)
    C False
    D True
    E False
    Ref. (*45a*) pp. 5–17

16. A True
    B True
    C False (asymptomatic
       or mildly pruritic)
    D True
    E True
    Ref. (*45b*) pp. 25–27

17. A False
    B True
    C True (because of
       dissection of air into
       pharangeal tissues)
    D False
    E True
    Ref. (*2*) p. 1270

18. A True
    B True (postictal)
    C True
    D True (especially in
       its early stages)
    E True
    Ref. (*28e*) pp. 280–283

19. A True (especially
       Lhermitte's sign)
    B False
    C True
    D True (carpal tunnel
       syndrome)
    E False
       (hyperventilation)
    Ref. (*28e*) pp. 334–335

20. A False
    B True
    C True
    D True
    E False
    Ref. (*46*)

21. A   True
     B   True
     C   False (phenformin)
     D   True
     E   False (bicarbonate
          infusion)
     Ref. (29) pp. 105–107

22. A   False (valvar type)
     B   False
     C   False
     D   True
     E   True
     Ref. (10) pp. 332–333

23. A   True (by producing
          the superior
          mediastinal
          syndrome)
     B   False
     C   True
     D   False
     E   False
     Ref. (10) p. 38

24. A   False
     B   False (an unusual
          finding)
     C   True
     D   True
     E   True
     Ref. (47) p. 271

25. A   True
     B   False
     C   False (associated
          with reduction in
          dose or stopping
          therapy)
     D   True
     E   True (very
          common)
     Ref. (47) p. 289

26. A   False
     B   True
     C   True
     D   True
     E   True
     Ref. (47) pp. 35–46

27. A   False
     B   True
     C   True
     D   True
     E   True
     Ref. (47)

28. A   False
     B   True
     C   True
     D   False
     E   True
     Ref. (47) p. 1146

29. A   False (usually
          associated with
          coexisting valvular
          disease)
     B   True
     C   True (berry
          aneurysms
          associated)
     D   True
     E   False
     Ref. (10) p. 319

30. A   True
     B   True
     C   True
     D   True
     E   False
     Ref. (4) p. 129

31. A False
     B True
     C False (also through
        the gastrointestinal
        tract)
     D True
     E True
     Ref. (*48*) pp. 1459–1466

32. A True
     B True
     C True
     D False
     E False
     Ref. (*20*) p. 215

33. A True
     B False
     C True
     D False
     E True
     Ref. (*20*) pp. 48–49

34. A True
     B False
     C False
     D False (crossed)
     E False (absent)
     Ref. (*26*) pp. 24–28

35. A True
     B True
     C True
     D True
     E False
     Ref. (*26*) pp. 435, 481, 483

36. A True
     B True
     C True
     D False
     E False (dementia)
     Ref. (*20*) pp. 121–122

37. A True
     B True
     C True
     D True
     E True
     Ref. (*28f*) pp. 413–424

38. A False
     B False (rapid
        intravenous
        injection)
     C True
     D False (works over 2
        hours)
     E False (produces
        paradoxical
        hypertension—use
        orally)
     Ref. (*28f*) pp. 453–454

39. A False (autosomal
        recessive)
     B False (autosomal
        dominant)
     C True
     D True
     E True
     Ref. (*28g*) p. 550

40. A True
     B False
        (hypoglycaemia)
     C True
     D True
     E False (staining of
        teeth)
     Ref. (*6*)

41. A   True
     B   False
     C   True
     D   True
     E   False
     Ref. (*28g*) pp. 565–573

42. A   False
     B   False (dominant)
     C   True
     D   True
     E   True
     Ref. (*28g*) p. 583

43. A   True
     B   False
     C   True
     D   False
     E   True
     Ref. (*28g*) p. 597

44. A   True
     B   True
     C   True
     D   True
     E   True
     Ref. (*28g*) p. 599

45. A   False
     B   True
     C   False
     D   True
     E   False
     Ref. (*28h*) p. 312

46. A   False
     B   True
     C   True
     D   True
     E   False
     Ref. (*28i*) p. 294

47. A   True
     B   True
     C   False
     D   False
     E   True
     Ref. (*28i*) p. 294

48. A   True
     B   True
     C   True
     D   True
     E   False
     Ref. (*28j*) p. 97

49. A   True
     B   True
     C   True
     D   True
     E   True
     Ref. (*28j*) p. 180

50. A   True
     B   False
         (predominantly
         associated with
         squamous
         carcinoma)
     C   False
     D   False (applies to
         adenocarcinoma)
     E   False·(seen in
         alveolar-cell
         carcinoma)
     Ref. (*50*) p. 175

51. A   False (rarely)
     B   True
     C   False
     D   True
     E   True
     Ref. (*51*)

52. A   True
    B   False (dead
        microfilariae
        provoke the
        response)
    C   True
    D   True
    E   False
    Ref. (2) pp. 897–898

53. A   True
    B   False
    C   False (occurs despite
        presence of
        antibodies)
    D   False (uncommon)
    E   False (idoxuridine,
        acycloguanisine,
        adenine arabinoside)
    Ref. (2) pp. 847–851

54. A   False (*Brucella
        abortus*)
    B   True
    C   True
    D   False (only
        sometimes)
    E   False (tetracyclines;
        streptomycin and
        sulphonamides in
        combination)
    Ref. (2) pp. 658–660

55. A   True
    B   True
    C   False
    D   True
    E   True (due to
        osteodystrophy)
    Ref. (2) pp. 1299–1307

56. A   False (7–10 days)
    B   True
    C   True
    D   False (raised white
        cell count)
    E   False
    Ref. (*33*)

57. A   True
    B   True
    C   True
    D   True
    E   True
    Ref. (*6*) p. 902

58. A   False
        (dihydropyridine
        derivative)
    B   True
    C   False
    D   True
    E   False
    Ref. (*54*)

59. A   False
    B   False
    C   True
    D   True
    E   True (some cases)
    Ref. (*4*) p. 246

60. A   True
    B   True
    C   False (it is the
        reverse)
    D   True
    E   False (to the right of
        the mode)
    Ref. (*17*)

Examination 6

(Time allotted: 2½ hours)

1. **Typical features of primary pulmonary hypertension are:**
    A   Central cyanosis
    B   Giant 'a' waves which appear later in the disease
    C   The occurrence of angina
    D   Congestive cardiac failure
    E   The unknown occurrence of sudden death

2. **In left ventricular failure:**
    A   Development of tricuspid incompetence relieves the pulmonary congestion
    B   Paroxysmal cardiac dyspnoea lasts for no more than 10–20 minutes
    C   The $Pa\text{CO}_2$ is increased if severe pulmonary oedema is present
    D   Effort dyspnoea always precedes orthopnoea and paroxysmal nocturnal dyspnoea
    E   The x-ray picture may be mistaken for a solid lung tumour

3. **The following statements are true regarding complete heart block:**
    A   It may develop during digitalis therapy
    B   Regular cannon 'a' waves are present
    C   The pulse is of small volume
    D   The first heart sound is soft
    E   A basal systolic murmur is usually present

111

4. **Cardiovascular syphilis:**
   A   Typically occurs after 1–3 years following exposure
   B   Directly involves the aortic cusps by the inflamma-tory process
   C   Commonly produces syphilitic myocarditis histo-logically
   D   Producing angina, often responds less effectively to nitroglycerine therapy
   E   May produce left ventricular aneurysm

5. **Clinical features of bronchiectasis include the fol-lowing:**
   A   In 75% of cases the symptoms are present by the 5th year of the onset of the disease
   B   Breathlessness on exertion is very common
   C   Associated chronic sinusitis is present in 70% of cases
   D   Almost all the patients are clubbed
   E   Central cyanosis is an early clinical sign

6. **Diffuse fibrosing alveolitis:**
   A   Is cryptogenic in the majority of the patients
   B   May be associated with chronic active hepatitis
   C   May follow therapy of chronic myeloid leukaemia
   D   Produces wheezing as a prominent feature
   E   Produces central cyanosis which is relieved by exer-cise

7. **A pleural effusion of 25g/litre (2.5g%) protein con-tent is characteristic of:**
   A   Meig's syndrome
   B   Myxoedema
   C   Chronic congestive heart failure
   D   Systemic lupus erythematosus
   E   Pulmonary infarction

8. **The following are true regarding coalworker's pneumoconiosis:**
   A Develops in miners after 1–5 years' exposure
   B The stage of simple pneumoconiosis is usually asymptomatic
   C Progressive massive fibrosis typically affects the lower lobes
   D Finger clubbing is common
   E Simple pneumoconiosis progresses even if further dust exposure is avoided

9. **The following are true regarding gastro-oesophageal reflux:**
   A It is determined by the competency of the lower oesophageal sphincter
   B The pain may simulate that of angina pectoris
   C Anticholinergic drugs are the medical treatment of choice
   D Where indicated fundoplication operations have given the best results
   E Weight loss should always be recommended in all patients

10. **In the postgastrectomy syndromes:**
    A Early dumping is due to rebound hypoglycaemia
    B Anaemia may be seen in up to 50% of cases
    C Anaemia is more common after gastroduodenostomy than after gastrojejunostomy
    D Folate deficiency is not uncommon
    E Patients may complain of severe backaches

11. **Tests useful in the diagnosis of malabsorption include:**
    A Oral glycine–1–14C glycocholate
    B Urinary indican
    C Serum carotene
    D D–Xylose test
    E Urinary 5-hydroxyindoleacetic acid

12. **In Crohn's disease:**
   A Presentation may resemble acute appendicitis
   B Diarrhoea with bright red bleeding is a frequent presentation
   C Renal failure may result
   D Acrocyanosis is common
   E Rectovaginal fistulas may occur

13. **Speech abnormalities are described in:**
   A Dementia paralytica (generalized paresis of the insane)
   B Congenital diplegia
   C Friedreich's ataxia
   D Amyotrophic lateral sclerosis
   E Severe glossitis

14. **Physiologically-elevated body temperature is found:**
   A In the tropics
   B Following a large meal
   C With emotional disturbances
   D During part of the menstrual cycle
   E Following the use of chlorpromazine

15. **An irregular liver edge is found in:**
   A Alcoholic cirrhosis where the patient has stopped drinking
   B Secondary syphilis
   C Hepatic actinomycosis
   D Wilson's disease
   E Amoebic dysentery

16. **Myoclonus may be caused by:**
   A Hypercalcaemia
   B Sodium valproate therapy
   C Disorders of the olivodentate system
   D Subacute sclerozing panencephalitis
   E Epilepsy

17. **Dystrophia myotonica is characterized by:**
    A   Progressive external ophthalmoplegia
    B   Cataracts
    C   Symptoms that may be found in childhood
    D   Fasciculations that are present early
    E   Tendon reflexes that are retained despite muscle wasting

18. **Claw feet deformities are seen with:**
    A   Wernicke's encephalopathy
    B   Charcot's arthropathy
    C   Syringomyelia
    D   Friedreich's ataxia
    E   Peroneal muscular atrophy

19. **Cerebrospinal fluid protein of 3 g/litre (300 mg%) is a finding in:**
    A   Beriberi polyneuritis
    B   General paresis of the insane
    C   Subdural haematoma
    D   Tuberculosis meningitis
    E   Congenital toxoplasmosis

20. **The following are seen in sickle-cell anaemia:**
    A   Dactylitis
    B   Retardation of secondary sexual characteristics
    C   Pathognomonic fundal changes
    D   Cardiac signs simulating mitral stenosis
    E   Normal urinary concentrating ability only if the sickle-cell trait is present

21. **In polycythaemia rubra vera:**
    A   The reticulocyte count is typically increased
    B   Leucocyte alkaline phosphatase score is low
    C   Hyperuricosuria is found in 30% of patients
    D   The capacity of the serum to bind vitamin B_{12} is increased
    E   Serum iron is characteristically raised

22. **The following statements are true about methaemoglobinaemia:**
   A   It is never associated with fatalities
   B   Blood has a characteristic chocolate-brown colour
   C   A positive family history may be elicited
   D   When treatment is indicated, intravenous methylene blue is the therapy of choice
   E   It is characterized by cyanosis

23. **In infantile eczema:**
   A   The rash is characteristically present at birth
   B   The papules are itchy
   C   Cold weather relieves the symptoms
   D   A family history of related disorders is elicited in 70% of cases
   E   White dermographism excludes the diagnosis

24. **Non-gonococcal urethritis:**
   A   Has an incubation period shorter than that of gonorrhoea
   B   Can be differentiated from gonorrhoea clinically
   C   Is commoner in white patients as opposed to black
   D   May be produced by ureaplasma urealyticum
   E   Must be treated with sulphonamides in high doses as the treatment of choice

25. **The following statements are true regarding Letterer–Siwe disease:**
   A   It is a slowly progressive disease of infancy
   B   Generalized lymphadenopathy is a common feature
   C   A severely purpuric rash may be present
   D   Most cases respond dramatically to corticosteroids
   E   'Honeycomb' appearances on x-ray are of diagnostic importance

26. **In tetralogy of Fallot:**
   A The pulmonic obstruction is valvar in most instances
   B Cyanosis may be absent in the first few months of life
   C Convulsions are a recognized association
   D The pulmonary second sound is widely split
   E Lung fields are typically plethoric

27. **Hepatic cirrhosis in childhood may be due to:**
   A Gaucher's disease
   B Veno-occlusive disease of the liver
   C Xanthomatosis
   D Maternal alcoholism during pregnancy
   E Coeliac disease

28. **At 12 weeks of age a normal child:**
   A Responds to name being called
   B Turns the head towards sound
   C Produces a grasp reflex on appropriate stimulation
   D Recognizes a feeding bottle placed before its eyes
   E Lifts its head from a pillow

29. **Korsakoff's syndrome is characterized by:**
   A Invariable finding of polyneuritis
   B A clear level of consciousness
   C Poor judgement
   D Anatomical changes in the hypothalamus
   E Confabulation

30. **Childhood schizophrenia is suggested by:**
   A Distortion in motility patterns
   B Persistent thumb sucking
   C Sustained resistance to changes in the environment
   D Infantile autism
   E Negativism

31. **Electroconvulsive therapy is indicated for:**
    A   Anorexia nervosa
    B   Severe depressive states
    C   Failure of response in a schizophrenic to medical treatment
    D   Severe uncontrollable status epilepticus
    E   A psychopath admitted following numerous crimes

32. **Favourable prognostic indicators in a schizophrenic include:**
    A   Acute onset of the illness
    B   A positive family history
    C   Stable previous personality
    D   A pyknic physique
    E   Early age of onset

33. **Haloperidol (Serenace):**
    A   Is effective in the treatment of depressive psychosis
    B   Has considerable antiemetic activity
    C   Has a high incidence of extrapyramidal side-effects
    D   Can be given by injection only
    E   May be used as a substitute for phenothiazines in patients developing jaundice after phenothiazine use

34. **The following drugs are antipyretic analgesics:**
    A   Colchicine
    B   Aspirin
    C   Phenacetin
    D   Amidopyrine
    E   Sulphinpyrazone

35. **Indications for penicillamine therapy include:**
    A   Systemic sclerosis
    B   Primary biliary cirrhosis
    C   Relapsing polychondritis
    D   Haemosiderosis
    E   Drug-induced chronic active hepatitis

36. **Side-effects of corticosteroids include:**
   A   Collagen loss
   B   Reduced leucocyte migration
   C   Avascular necrosis of bones
   D   Hypercalcaemia
   E   Increased vascular permeability

37. **Digitalis therapy:**
   A   Is contraindicated in atrial tachycardia
   B   Should be discontinued prior to attempted cardioversion
   C   Is likely to produce toxicity in the presence of hyperkalaemia
   D   Is contraindicated in cor pulmonale
   E   Is beneficial in hypertrophic obstructive cardiomyopathy

38. **Polydactyly is described with:**
   A   Laurence–Moon–Biedl syndrome
   B   Marfan's syndrome
   C   Turner's syndrome
   D   Fanconi's congenital aplastic anaemia
   E   Ventricular septal defect

39. **An opening snap may be found in:**
   A   Mitral stenosis due to rheumatic heart disease
   B   Congenital mitral stenosis
   C   Mitral incompetence associated with a rigid posterior valve leaflet but a normal anterior leaflet
   D   Left atrial myxoma
   E   Severe aortic incompetence

40. **The following are true regarding acromegaly:**
   A   Patients may complain of nocturnal paraesthesiae in the hands
   B   Marked skin dryness is a prominent feature
   C   Female patients may complain of increasing limb and body hair
   D   Impotence is common in the male
   E   The diagnosis cannot be made if the pituitary fossa is of normal size on skull x-ray

41. **The treatment of thyrotoxic crisis includes:**
   A High doses of intravenous hydrocortisone
   B Keeping the patient warm
   C Administration of beta blocking agents
   D Immediate administration of carbimazole
   E Administration of iodide

42. **Features of glucagonoma include the following:**
   A It is a tumour of the beta cells of the islets of Langerhans
   B It typically produces necrolytic migratory erythema
   C Many of these tumours are malignant
   D It may produce mild diabetes mellitus
   E Treatment includes total gastrectomy

43. **Specific indications for dialysis include:**
   A A serum potassium of 7.4 mmol/litre (7.4 mEq/litre)
   B A blood pH of 7.2
   C A blood urea of 63 mmol/litre (378 mg/100 ml)
   D Presence of pericarditis
   E Severe left renal angle tenderness

44. **Renal arterial infarction:**
   A Is almost always symptomatic
   B Tenderness is present in the affected loin
   C Hypertension may develop
   D A radioactive renogram is indicated
   E Embolectomy is of no value

45. **The renal physiological changes in pregnancy include:**
   A Decrease in the glomerular filtration rate
   B Decrease in the blood urea to 2.5–3.3 mmol/litre (15–20 mg/100 ml)
   C Glycosuria found in almost all patients
   D Development of lactosuria in early pregnancy
   E Increases uric acid clearance

46. **Myalgias are typical of:**
   A Thomsen's disease (congenital myotonia)
   B Myoglobinuria
   C Progressive muscular dystrophy
   D Renal tubular acidosis
   E McArdle's syndrome

47. **In Paget's disease of bone (osteitis deformans):**
   A The serum alkaline phosphatase is normal unless a fracture is present
   B The serum phosphorous is typically low
   C Renal calculi are common
   D High dose steroids are the treatment of choice
   E Heel pad thickness is classically increased

48. **In Hodgkin's disease:**
   A Delayed hypersensitivity is impaired
   B Needle biopsy of the bone marrow discloses the diagnosis in 50% of cases
   C Eosinophilia is present in 10% of cases
   D An absolute lymphocytosis is typical
   E Haemolytic anaemia may develop

49. **Severe irradiation produces:**
   A An increased incidence of leukaemia
   B Thrombocytopenia which begins in about four days
   C An increased incidence of visceral malignancy
   D Leukaemoid reactions in some patients
   E Haemolytic anaemia

50. **With regards to transplant immunology:**
   A Hyperacute rejection is mediated by T-cell lymphocytes
   B Early acute rejection is mediated by B lymphocytes
   C Chronic rejection is immunoglobulin mediated
   D Steroids are lymphocytotoxic and very effective in reversing acute rejection of a donor organ
   E Antilymphocyte globulin is effective

51. **Homocystinuria:**
    A Is autosomal dominant
    B Is due to cystothionine synthetase absence
    C Patients have ectopia lentis
    D Carries a higher incidence of arterial and venous occlusions
    E Has a higher incidence of renal calculi

52. **In bromism:**
    A The patient may present with psychosis
    B Blood levels of bromine may be normal
    C Cerebrospinal fluid protein is increased in acute bromide poisoning
    D The serum chloride may be disproportionately raised
    E Typical skin lesions may be found

53. **Osteoporosis:**
    A Produces a raised serum calcium
    B Typically produces an elevated alkaline phosphatase
    C May produce bone pain
    D Is improved by bed rest
    E Responds well to modern therapy

54. **Bicarbonate=18 mmol/litre (18 mEq/litre), Potassium=6.5 mmol/litre (6.5 mEq/litre), Sodium= 111 mmol/litre (111 mEq/litre), Chloride=72 mmol/litre (72 mEq/litre), pH=7.2. These results are compatible with:**
    A Cholera
    B Severe diabetic ketoacidosis
    C Addison's disease
    D Severe vomiting
    E Gastrocolic fistula

55. **With regards to the Philadelphia (Ph$_1$) chromosome, the following are true:**
   A   In chronic myeloid leukaemia following therapy, the Ph$_1$ cell line disappears from the blood but persists in the marrow
   B   It has been detected only in the erythroblasts
   C   The Ph$_1$ negative form of chronic myeloid leukaemia rarely has a white cell count over 100 000/ mm^3
   D   The Ph$_1$ negative form has a better response to chemotherapy
   E   Is the karyotype abnormality found in the majority of cases of chronic myeloid leukaemia

56. **Mydriasis is found in:**
   A   Oculomotor nerve paralysis
   B   Horner's syndrome
   C   Retrobulbar neuritis
   D   Iritis
   E   Holmes–Adie pupil syndrome

57. **The following statements are true regarding rubella in pregnancy:**
   A   It carries a risk to the fetus in the first trimester
   B   Coarctation of the aorta commonly results in the newborn
   C   Deafness occurs in the newborn
   D   The child may develop a retinopathy
   E   The virus can readily be isolated from the throat of the infected newborn whether or not signs of the disease are present

58. **Complications of measles include:**
   A   Common occurrence of severe corneal ulceration
   B   Cancrum oris
   C   Higher incidence of acute appendicitis
   D   Post-measles encephalomyelopathy one month later
   E   Subacute sclerosing panencephalitis years after attack of measles

59. **Specific contraindications to routine primary vaccination include:**
   A   Pregnancy, only in the first trimester
   B   Infantile eczema
   C   Immunosuppressive therapy
   D   Under six months of age
   E   During an epidemic

60. **The following statements are true:**
   A   The geometric mean is always less in value than the arithmetic mean
   B   The arithmetic mean is the measure to be preferred in data which is symmetrically distributed
   C   The median is also called the measure of central value
   D   The standard deviation is a poor measure of dispersion
   E   The value of the variable which occurs with the least frequency is the mode

42°/.

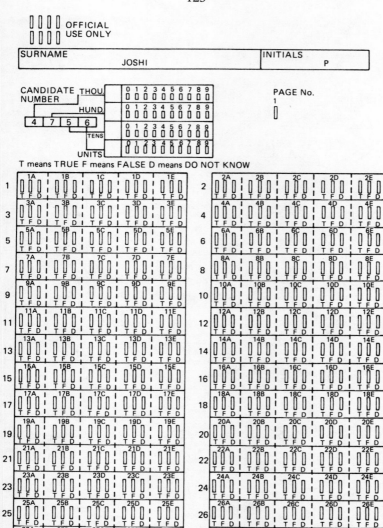

OFFICIAL USE ONLY

SURNAME JOSHI

INITIALS P

CANDIDATE NUMBER

4 7 5 6

THOU. 0 1 2 3 4 5 6 7 8 9
HUND. 0 1 2 3 4 5 6 7 8 9
TENS 0 1 2 3 4 5 6 7 8 9
UNITS 0 1 2 3 4 5 6 7 8 9

PAGE No. 1

T means TRUE F means FALSE D means DO NOT KNOW

126

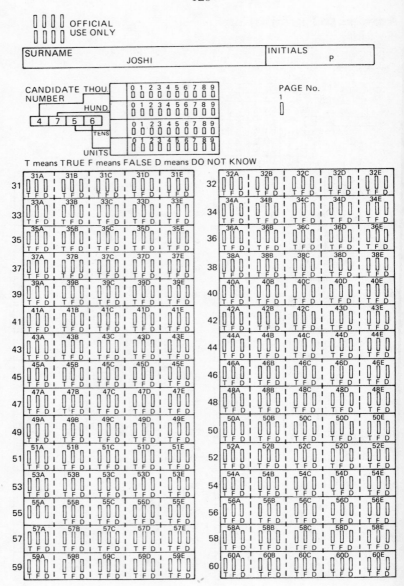

OFFICIAL USE ONLY

SURNAME JOSHI

INITIALS P

CANDIDATE NUMBER 4 7 5 6

PAGE No. 1

T means TRUE F means FALSE D means DO NOT KNOW

Answers to Examination 6

(For complete References see Chapter 3)

1. A   False (absent)
    B   False (early)
    C   True (occasionally)
    D   True
    E   False (not uncommon)
    Ref. (*10*) pp. 577–580

2. A   True
    B   True
    C   False
    D   False
    E   True (vanishing tumour)
    Ref. (*10*) pp. 234–236

3. A   True
    B   False (irregular)
    C   False (collapsing)
    D   False (variable intensity)
    E   True
    Ref. (*10*) p. 215

4. A   False (15–25 years)
    B   False (therefore there is no aortic stenosis found)
    C   False
    D   True
    E   True
    Ref. (*10*) pp. 549–554

5. A   True
    B   False
    C   True
    D   False (about 50%)
    E   False
    Ref. (*9*) pp. 114–121

6. A   True
    B   True
    C   True (Busulphan)
    D   False
    E   False
    Ref. (*9*) pp. 237–241

7. A   False
    B   False
    C   False
    D   True
    E   True
    Ref. (*9*) p. 244

8. A   False (after 20 years' exposure)
    B   True
    C   False (upper)
    D   False
    E   False
    Ref. (*9*) pp. 228–229

9. A   True
    B   True
    C   False
    D   True
    E   False
    Ref. (*2*) pp. 1366–1367

10. A   False
    B   True
    C   False (reverse)
    D   False (rare)
    E   True (osteomalacia)
    Ref. (*2*) p. 1381

11. A True
     B True
     C True
     D True
     E True
     Ref. (2) pp. 1396–1399

12. A True
     B False
     C True (due to amyloidosis)
     D True
     E True
     Ref. (2) pp. 1411–1416

13. A True (slurred speech)
     B True (slurred speech)
     C True (scanning speech)
     D True (dysarthria)
     E True (dysarthria)
     Ref. (24) pp. 288–292

14. A True
     B True
     C True (especially in children)
     D True (at ovulation)
     E False (decreases the temperature)
     Ref. (32) p. 116

15. A True (this leads to the development of macronodular cirrhosis)
     B False (tertiary form)
     C True
     D False
     E False
     Ref. (24) pp. 269–270

16. A False
     B False
     C True
     D True
     E True
     Ref. (26) p. 75

17. A False (ocular muscular dystrophy)
     B True
     C True
     D False
     E False
     Ref. (26) p. 382

18. A False
     B False
     C True
     D True
     E True
     Ref. (26) p. 454

19. A False
     B True
     C False
     D True
     E True
     Ref. (4) pp. 172–174

20. A True
     B True
     C False
     D True (see Harrison's 7th edition, pp. 1620–1621)
     E False
     Ref. (2) pp. 1547–1550

21. A False
     B False (high)
     C True
     D True
     E False
     Ref. (2) pp. 1576–1579

22. A   False
     B   True
     C   True
     D   True
     E   True
     Ref. (2) pp. 1551–1552

23. A   False (3rd–4th
         month)
     B   True
     C   False (aggravates)
     D   True
     E   False
     Ref. (3) p. 47

24. A   False (1–3 weeks)
     B   False
     C   True
     D   True
     E   False
     Ref. (46) pp. 1–2, 12

25. A   False (rapidly
         progressive)
     B   True
     C   True
     D   False (only some do)
     E   True
     Ref. (15) p. 210

26. A   False (infundibular)
     B   True
     C   True
     D   False (single)
     E   False
     Ref. (15) p. 288

27. A   True
     B   True
     C   True
     D   False
     E   False
     Ref. (15) pp. 340–341

28. A   False (6 months)
     B   True
     C   False (4 weeks)
     D   True
     E   False (6 months)
     Ref. (15)

29. A   False
     B   True
     C   True
     D   False (periventri-
         cular and
         periaqueductal
         grey matter and
         mamillary bodies
     E   True
     Ref. (35) p. 236

30. A   True
     B   False
     C   True
     D   False
     E   False
     Ref. (35) p. 278

31. A   False
     B   True
     C   True
     D   False
     E   False
     Ref. (35) pp. 314–315

32. A   True
     B   False (of little value)
     C   True
     D   True
     E   False (poor
         prognosis)
     Ref. (35) p. 179

33. A   False (excited)
     B   True
     C   True
     D   False (orally)
     E   True
     Ref. (56) pp. 289, 306

34. A   False
     B   True
     C   True
     D   True
     E   False
     Ref. (56) pp. 353–362

35. A   True
     B   True
     C   False
     D   True
     E   False
     Ref. (57) p. 254

36. A   True
     B   True
     C   True
     D   False
     E   False
     Ref. (1) p. 177

37. A   False (in ventricular
             tachycardia)
     B   True
     C   False (hypokalaemia)
     D   False
     E   False
     Ref. (56) pp. 117–182

38. A   True
     B   False
     C   True
     D   False
     E   True
     Ref. (58) p. 167

39. A   True
     B   True (a rare
             malformation)
     C   True
     D   True (in 10%
             because of markedly
             increased left atrial
             pressure–the snap is
             usually soft and late)
     E   False
     Ref. (58) p. 260

40. A   True
     B   False (sweaty)
     C   True
     D   True
     E   False
     Ref. (16) p. 5

41. A   False
     B   False (cool the
             patient)
     C   True
     D   True
     E   True
     Ref. (16) p. 62

42. A   False (alpha cells)
     B   True
     C   True
     D   True
     E   False
     Ref. (16) p. 176

43. A   True
     B   False (less than 7.15)
     C   True (in acute renal
             failure)
     D   True
     E   False (look for the
             cause)
     Ref. (5) pp. 104–105

44. A   False
   B   True
   C   True
   D   True
   E   False
   Ref. (5) p. 141

45. A   False (increases)
   B   True
   C   False (in about 40%)
   D   False (in late pregnancy)
   E   True
   Ref. (5) p. 159

46. A   False
   B   True
   C   False
   D   True
   E   True
   Ref. (4) p. 191

47. A   False (markedly elevated)
   B   False (normal)
   C   True
   D   False
   E   False (in acromegaly)
   Ref. (4) p. 196

48. A   True
   B   False (5% at the time of diagnosis)
   C   True
   D   False (consider another diagnosis)
   E   True
   Ref. (2) pp. 1635–1641

49. A   True
   B.   True (4–7 days)
   C   True (e.g. liver cancer)
   D   True
   E   False
   Ref. (4) pp. 212–213

50. A   False (preformed antibodies)
   B   False (T lymphocytes)
   C   True
   D   True
   E   True
   Ref. (5) pp. 18–19

51. A   False (autosomal recessive)
   B   True
   C   True
   D   True
   E   False (homocystine is soluble in urine)
   Ref. (2) pp. 463–468

52. A   True
   B   False (increases)
   C   True
   D   True
   E   True
   Ref. (4) p. 388

53. A   False (normal serum calcium)
   B   False (unless an associated fracture is present)
   C   True
   D   False
   E   False
   Ref. (8) pp. 975–977

54. A   False (the potassium is decreased)
   B   False (bicarbonate levels are much lower)
   C   True
   D   False (develop alkalosis)
   E   False
   Ref. (4) p. 255

55. A   True
    B   False
    C   True
    D   False
    E   True
    Ref. (*8*) pp. 357–358

56. A   True
    B   False (small)
    C   True
    D   True
    E   True
    Ref. (*24*) pp. 274–275

57. A   True
    B   False
    C   True
    D   True
    E   True
    Ref. (*8*) pp. 135–137

58. A   False (very rare—
        may lead to
        blindness)
    B   True
    C   True
    D   False (5–10 days
        later)
    E   True
    Ref. (*8*) pp. 138–139

59. A   False
    B   True
    C   True
    D   False
    E   False
    Ref. (*8*) p. 132

60. A   True
    B   True
    C   True
    D   False
    E   False (greatest
        frequency)
    Ref. (*17*)

Examination 7

(Time allotted 2½ hours)

1. **Deficiency of alpha$_1$ antitrypsin enzyme is associated with:**
   - A   A positive family history of emphysema
   - B   An early onset of exertional dyspnoea
   - C   A restrictive lung defect
   - D   Bullae in the upper and middle lobes
   - E   Gastrointestinal malabsorption

2. **Recurrent pneumonia is caused by:**
   - A   Chronic alcoholism
   - B   Multiple myeloma
   - C   Sickle-cell anaemia
   - D   Oesophageal lesions
   - E   Allergic bronchopulmonary aspergillosis

3. **Non-infective pneumonia is described:**
   - A   Post-irradiation
   - B   With chronic corticosteroid administration
   - C   With accidental ingestion of kerosene
   - D   With schistosomiasis
   - E   With use of nose drops

4. **Causes of a solitary pulmonary 'coin' lesion include:**
   A   Rheumatoid arthritis
   B   Bronchopneumonia
   C   Arteriovenous fistula
   D   Hydatid cyst
   E   Hodgkin's disease

5. **With continued administration, barbiturates:**
   A   Precipitate convulsions
   B   Produce physical dependence
   C   Produce voluntary muscle relaxation
   D   Produce parkinsonism
   E   Produce ataxia

6. **Aminocaproic acid is used in the treatment of:**
   A   Waldenström's macroglobulinaemia
   B   Subarachnoid haemorrhage
   C   Abruptio placentae
   D   Haemophilia
   E   Antithrombin III deficiency

7. **Megaloblastic anaemia may occur:**
   A   In patients receiving carbamazepine (Tegretol)
   B   In patients receiving primidone (Mysoline)
   C   In patients receiving methotrexate
   D   In patients receiving co-trimoxazole (Bactrim)
   E   In patients with ulcerative colitis

8. **Hypoglycaemic attacks associated with sulphonylurea therapy are potentiated by:**
   A   Probenecid
   B   Phenylbutazone
   C   Bishydroxycoumarin
   D   Monoamine oxidase inhibitors
   E   Salicylates

9.   **The following statements are true:**
A   Carbenoxolone (Biogastrone) has a demonstrated beneficial effect on duodenal ulcers
B   Oestrogens improve the course of gastric ulcers in males
C   Aluminium hydroxide gel is used in large doses to increase calcium absorption in uraemia
D   Magnesium salts used as antacids may produce constipation
E   After antacid ingestion, action usually persists for up to six hours

10.   **In uncomplicated rheumatic fever the following are recognized:**
A   Clubbing of the fingers
B   Pleurisy
C   Anaemia
D   Splenomegaly
E   Microscopic haematuria

11.   **In constrictive pericarditis:**
A   Ascites is often out of proportion to the degree of dependent oedema
B   Pedal oedema is a prominent feature in chronic cases
C   Pleuritic pain may be present
D   A pansystolic murmur which increases on inspiration is characteristic
E   Prominent 'v' waves in the neck are present

12.   **In atrial septal defects:**
A   Patients are usually symptomatic by the second decade
B   Atrial fibrillation occurs
C   Pulmonary systolic thrill may be present
D   The murmur is produced by flow across the defect
E   A mid–diastolic murmur increasing on expiration is characteristic

13. **In fat embolism:**
   A   Petechial haemorrhages in the skin are rare
   B   Cyanosis is present
   C   Convulsions are usually ominous
   D   Intravenous alcohol is the treatment of choice
   E   Haemoptysis may occur

14. **Neurological manifestations of myxoedema include:**
   A   Optic atrophy
   B   Paraesthesiae in the hands
   C   Cerebellar signs
   D   Loss of vibration sense in the feet
   E   Deafness

15. **A diabetic patient may present for the first time with:**
   A   Increasing weight
   B   Peripheral vascular disease
   C   Retinal detachment
   D   Oculomotor nerve palsy
   E   Severe pruritis

16. **In cystic fibrosis the following are characteristic:**
   A   Decreased sweat chloride levels
   B   Anorexia
   C   Cirrhosis of the liver
   D   Chronic paranasal sinusitis
   E   Absent pancreatic enzymes on aspiration of duodenal contents

17. **Carcinoma of the gall bladder:**
   A   Is common in males
   B   May be associated with gall-stones in up to 90% of cases
   C   Almost never produces an enlarged liver
   D   Very rarely produces distant metastases
   E   Commonly arises from an adenomatous polyp

18. **The following features are typical of Whipple's disease:**
    A   It occurs predominantly in young adults
    B   Polyserositis
    C   Lymphadenopathy
    D   PAS-positive material on jejunal biopsy
    E   Dramatic complete response to tetracyclines given in doses of 1 g daily in divided doses for 3 weeks

19. **Diarrhoea in diabetes:**
    A   Is usually severe and explosive
    B   May contain gross blood in the stool
    C   Is associated with an abnormal radiological small-intestinal pattern
    D   Should be treated with anticholinergic drugs as the treatment of choice
    E   Is usually progressive in severity

20. **Recognized causes of impotence include:**
    A   Multiple sclerosis
    B   Androgen deficiency
    C   Tabes dorsalis
    D   Parietal lobe lesions
    E   Malignant hypertension

21. **Bilateral external ophthalmoplegia of sudden onset occurs with:**
    A   Botulism
    B   Myasthenia gravis
    C   Wernicke's encephalopathy
    D   Neurosyphilis
    E   Diphtheria

22. **In paroxysmal myoglobinuria the following are true:**
    A   Absence of erythrocytes in the urine
    B   Severe muscle weakness
    C   Renal failure may result
    D   Approximately 50% of patients die in the acute attack
    E   McArdle's disease is a cause

23. **The following are true regarding acute transverse myelitis:**
A   It may occur as an initial event in multiple sclerosis
B   Vibration sense is preserved
C   Bladder dysfunction is always transient
D   The motor disorder is supranuclear in type
E   Complete recovery never occurs

24. **Platybasia:**
A   May be caused by rickets
B   May present with loss of proprioception
C   May be associated with syringomyelia
D   Has no therapy of any value
E   Characteristically produces low intracranial pressure

25. **Factors directly concerned with concentrating urine under physiological conditions include:**
A   Circulating antidiuretic hormone
B   The blood pressure
C   Normal tubular response
D   Potassium deficiency
E   Pyrexial illness

26. **In nephrotic syndrome:**
A   Prognosis is better in males than in females
B   Malignant hypertension may occur
C   Intermittent microscopic haematuria regularly implies advancing parenchymal destruction
D   Renal biopsy is of great value in assessing prognosis
E   Treatment of the initiating condition is rarely successful

27. **The adult form of polycystic kidneys:**
A   Has an autosomal recessive inheritance
B   Always has proteinuria present
C   Commonly has malignant hypertension
D   May present with polycythaemia
E   Shows characteristic changes on intravenous pyelogram

28. **In infective endocarditis:**
   A   Bacteria are commonly found in the kidney
   B   Renal lesions may be due to an abnormal antibody
        —antigen response
   C   Frank haematuria should suggest an unrelated cause
   D   Renal involvement adversely affects the final out-
        come
   E   Persistent hypocomplementaemia is the rule

29. **In acute pyelonephritis:**
   A   Shaking chills are characteristic
   B   Diarrhoea may occur
   C   Absence of loin pains excludes the diagnosis
   D   An intravenous pyelogram is of no value in the
        diagnosis
   E   Blood cultures should be done routinely to confirm
        the diagnosis

30. **The following immunoglobulin changes are char-
    acteristic:**
   A   Acute viral hepatitis produces a monoclonal gamm-
        opathy
   B   Increased IgG and IgA are common in Laënnec's
        cirrhosis
   C   IgG is strikingly elevated in chronic active hepatitis
   D   Increased IgA is invariable in primary hepatoma
   E   IgM is increased in primary biliary cirrhosis

31. **Splenectomy may be beneficial in:**
   A   Hereditary spherocytosis
   B   Idiopathic thrombocytopenia purpura
   C   Sickle-cell anaemia
   D   Thalassaemia major
   E   Paroxysmal nocturnal haemoglobinuria

32. **Paroxysmal cold haemoglobinuria is associated
    with:**
   A   Aching pains in the back
   B   Haemolysis occurring at low temperatures
   C   A strongly positive direct antiglobin (Coombs) test
   D   Congenital syphilis
   E   A positive Donath—Landsteiner test

33. **Sickle-cell anaemia:**
   A   Is almost entirely confined to negroes
   B   Is associated with sudden attacks of severe abdominal pains
   C   The anaemia is usually mild
   D   Osmotic fragility is increased
   E   Pregnancy is contraindicated

34. **Features of the lateral medullary syndrome include:**
   A   Contralateral ataxia
   B   Ipsilateral Horner's syndrome
   C   Hoarseness
   D   Diplopia
   E   Visual field defects

35. **In acute idiopathic polyneuritis:**
   A   Weakness involves the proximal as well as the distal muscles
   B   Pain is common
   C   Paraesthesiae are frequent
   D   Retention of urine occurs
   E   Lymphadenopathy occurs

36. **Pellagra:**
   A   Produces mental symptoms in up to 70% of patients
   B   Is caused by excessive ingestion of corn
   C   May run an acute course and be fatal
   D   Produces delirium as the most frequent mental symptom
   E   Responds to therapy only 1 week after commencing therapy

37. **The following are recognized hallucinogens:**
   A   Cannabis
   B   Cocaine
   C   Lysergic acid diethylamide
   D   Chloral hydrate
   E   Suramin

38. **There is a higher incidence of suicide in:**
   A   Depressive psychosis
   B   Psychopaths
   C   Obsessive-compulsive neurosis
   D   Chronic alcoholism
   E   Epileptics

39. **The following features suggest that amnesia is of psychogenic origin:**
   A   Associated impairment of intellectual function
   B   A selective amnesia for inconvenient events
   C   Sudden and complete recovery of memory
   D   Generalized loss of memory for recent and remote events
   E   Perseveration

40. **Features of Hand–Schueller–Christian disease include:**
   A   Diabetes insipidus
   B   Exophthalmos
   C   Hypercholesterolaemia
   D   Xanthoma disseminatum
   E   Lipaemia retinalis

41. **Cerebral palsy may present with:**
   A   Hypotonia
   B   Ataxia
   C   Athetosis
   D   Bitemporal hemianopia
   E   Flapping tremor

42. **Contraindications to breast-feeding include:**
   A   Thyrotoxicosis
   B   Maternal tuberculosis
   C   Disseminated sclerosis
   D   Puerperal psychosis
   E   Pneumococcal pneumonia

43. **With regards to viral hepatitis in children:**
   A   Virus B is the commonest cause
   B   Cirrhosis of the liver is a common sequel
   C   Pruritis is uncommon in children
   D   Splenomegaly is commoner than in adults
   E   Acute liver failure is rare

44. **A type II (cytotoxic) hypersensitivity reaction is seen in:**
   A   Poison ivy allergy
   B   Post-streptococcal glomerulonephritis
   C   Rheumatic fever
   D   Penicillin allergy
   E   Chronic mucocutaneous candidiasis

45. **Immunosuppressive therapy is of value in:**
   A   Psoriatic arthritis
   B   Regional ileitis (Crohn's disease)
   C   Adult nephrotic syndrome
   D   Rheumatoid arthritis
   E   Multiple sclerosis

46. **Complications of diphtheria include:**
   A   Diaphragmatic paralysis
   B   Airways obstruction
   C   Bronchopulmonary diphtheria
   D   Glossopharangeal neuritis
   E   Subacute sclerosing panencephalitis

47. **Tetanus:**
   A   Is caused by an anaerobic Gram-positive rod
   B   Organism is found in the intestinal tract of man
   C   Produces carpopedal spasms
   D   Patients are mentally confused on admission
   E   May produce paralytic ileus

48. **In primary tuberculosis:**
   A   The majority of the lesions are in the lower two-thirds of the lung
   B   Bilateral hilar adenopathy is common in the adolescent
   C   Miliary tuberculosis may develop
   D   Phlyctenular conjunctivitis is characteristic
   E   Erythema nodosum does not occur

49. **Tropical eosinophilia:**
   A   May present with asthma
   B   Is commonly accompanied by false positive serological tests for syphilis
   C   Produces a high titre of cold agglutinins
   D   May be produced by diethylcarbamazine therapy
   E   May present with recurrent haemoptysis

50. ***Trichinella spiralis* is characterized by:**
   A   Prodromal diarrhoea in adults
   B   Severe muscle pains
   C   Periorbital oedema
   D   Subconjunctival haemorrhages
   E   Splinter haemorrhages in the nails

51. **Myopathy typically occurs in:**
   A   Central core disease
   B   McArdle's syndrome
   C   Strychnine poisoning
   D   Thomsen's disease
   E   Hypothyroidism

52. **Silicosis:**
   A   Usually has a short latent period
   B   Has a high incidence of scleroderma
   C   Has an increased incidence of bronchogenic carcinoma
   D   Produces characteristic calcification of the hilar glands
   E   An obstructive defect on lung function tests is present

53. **Bullous skin lesions are found in:**
   A   Dermatitis herpetiformis
   B   Barbiturate toxicity
   C   Albright's disease
   D   Ataxia telengiectasia
   E   Pemphigoid

54. **Galactosaemia is characterized by:**
   A   Cirrhosis
   B   Mental retardation
   C   Cataracts only if due to galactokinase deficiency
   D   Improvement following the use of soya bean preparations
   E   Cataracts present at birth

55. **Spontaneous hypoglycaemia typically occurs in:**
   A   Primary hepatoma
   B   Pancreatic islet–cell tumour
   C   Thiazide toxicity
   D   Tolbutamide therapy
   E   Thyrotoxicosis

56. **The following blood changes are compatible with a diagnosis of Hodgkin's disease:**
   A   Leucoerythroblastic anaemia
   B   Reticulocyte count of 15%
   C   Leucocytosis
   D   Thrombocytosis
   E   Eosinophilia

57. **Trichomoniasis:**
   A   Produces perianal intertrigo
   B   Is transmitted by sexual intercourse
   C   May produce marked systemic effects
   D   May be completely asymptomatic
   E   Is a commonly acquired infection in the newborn from an infected mother

58. **Band–keratopathy occurs in:**
   A   Behçet's disease
   B   Wilson's disease
   C   Vitamin D intoxication
   D   Hypoparathyroidism
   E   Sarcoidosis

59. **The patient with Adie's pupil:**
   A   Is typically asymptomatic
   B   Has one pupil larger than the other
   C   Shows resistance in response to 2.5% mecholyl in the affected eye
   D   Must have serology done to exclude tabes dorsalis
   E   May have brisk ankle jerks

60. **The following statements are true:**
   A   The standard deviation may be a negative value
   B   The value of the standard error depends upon the sample size and the standard deviation of the population
   C   By significance is meant that an observed result is likely to have arisen by chance
   D   The mode is usually the same in value as the median
   E   In a positively skewed distribution, the median is greater than the mode but less than the mean

146

SURNAME		INITIALS	
	JOSHI		P

CANDIDATE NUMBER THOU.

| 0 1 2 3 4 5 6 7 8 9 |
| ▯▯▯▯▯▯▯▯▯▯ |

HUND.

| 0 1 2 3 4 5 6 7 8 9 |
| ▯▯▯▯▯▯▯▯▯▯ |

| 4 | 7 | 5 | 6 |

TENS

| 0 1 2 3 4 5 6 7 8 9 |
| ▯▯▯▯▯▯▯▯▯▯ |

UNITS

| 0 1 2 3 4 5 6 7 8 9 |
| ▯▯▯▯▯▯▯▯▯▯ |

PAGE No.
1
▯

T means TRUE F means FALSE D means DO NOT KNOW

147

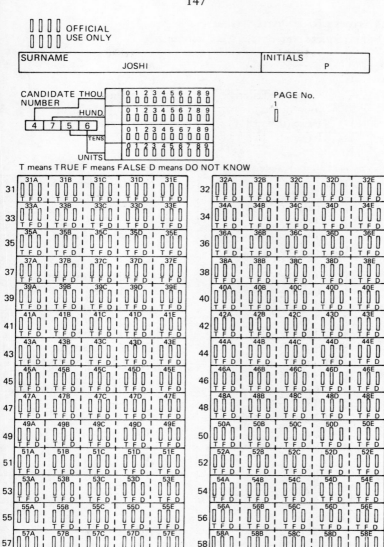

SURNAME
JOSHI

INITIALS
P

CANDIDATE NUMBER

THOU. 0 1 2 3 4 5 6 7 8 9
HUND. 0 1 2 3 4 5 6 7 8 9
4 7 5 6
TENS 0 1 2 3 4 5 6 7 8 9
UNITS 0 1 2 3 4 5 6 7 8 9

PAGE No.
1

T means TRUE F means FALSE D means DO NOT KNOW

Answers to Examination 7

(For complete References see Chapter 3)

1. A True
    B True
    C False (obstructive
       lung defect)
    D False (lower lobes)
    E False
    Ref. (9) p. 150

2. A True
    B True
    C False
    D True
    E True
    Ref. (9) p. 96

3. A True
    B False
    C True
    D True
    E True
    Ref. (9) p. 97

4. A True
    B False
    C True
    D True
    E False
    Ref. (9) p. 190

5. A False
    B True
    C True
    D False
    E True
    Ref. (7) p. 202

6. A False
    B True
    C True
    D True
    E False
    Ref. (7) p. 162

7. A True
    B True
    C True
    D True
    E False
    Ref. (7) pp. 422–423

8. A True
    B True
    C True
    D True
    E True
    Ref. (7) p. 341

9. A False (gastric ulcers)
    B False (duodenal
       ulcers)
    C False (impairs
       phosphate
       absorption)
    D False (frequent liquid
       motions are
       produced)
    E False (antacid action
       persists for 1–3
       hours)
    Ref. (7) pp. 290–291

10. A True
    B True
    C True
    D True
    E True
    Ref. (10) pp. 368, 414

11. A True
    B False (in active cases)
    C True
    D False
    E False
    Ref. (10) pp. 454–459

12. A False
     B True
     C True
     D False
     E False (increases on
        inspiration)
     Ref. (*10*) pp. 288–289

13. A False (characteristic)
     B True
     C True
     D False (of no value)
     E True
     Ref. (*10*) p. 575

14. A False
     B True
     C True
     D False
     E True (in the
        congenital or
        acquired type)
     Ref. (*16*) p. 64

15. A True (especially if
        steroid-induced)
     B True
     C True
     D True
     E True
     Ref. (*16*) p. 116

16. A False (increased
        levels are found)
     B False (increase in
        appetite)
     C True
     D True
     E True
     Ref. (*59*) pp. 387–388

17. A False (F:M: :3:1)
     B True
     C False
     D False (60% at time of
        operation)
     E False (rare)
     Ref. (*59*) p. 766

18. A False (4th–7th
        decades)
     B True
     C True
     D True
     E False (may have to
        continue
        indefinitely)
     Ref. (*59*) p. 696

19. A True
     B True (rarely)
     C False
     D False (ineffective)
     E False
     Ref. (*59*) p. 1063

20. A True
     B True
     C True
     D False (temporal lobe
        lesions)
     E False
     Ref. (*59*) p. 1253

21. A True
     B True
     C True (owing to
        thiamine deficiency)
     D False
     E False
     Ref. (*59*) p. 2154

22. A   True
    B   True
    C   True
    D   False (15%)
    E   True
    Ref. (59) p. 2179

23. A   True
    B   False
    C   False
    D   True
    E   False
    Ref. (59) pp. 2106, 2108

24. A   True
    B   True
    C   True
    D   False
    E   False
    Ref. (59) p. 2135

25. A   True
    B   False
    C   True
    D   True
    E   True
    Ref. (34) pp. 58–61

26. A   False (the reverse)
    B   True
    C   False
    D   False
    E   True
    Ref. (34) pp. 147–150

27. A   False
    B   True
    C   False
    D   True
    E   True
    Ref. (34) pp. 401–404

28. A   False (almost never)
    B   True
    C   False
    D   False
    E   False
    Ref. (34) pp. 288–290

29. A   True
    B   True
    C   False
    D   False
    E   False
    Ref. (2) pp. 1327–1331

30. A   False
    B   True
    C   True
    D   False
    E   True
    Ref. (2) pp. 317–319
    Ref. (59) pp. 1894,
    1469–1470

31. A   True
    B   True
    C   False
    D   False
    E   False
    Ref. (2) pp. 1542, 1556,
    1557

32. A   True
    B   False (haemolysin
        unites with the red
        cells at low
        temperatures)
    C   True
    D   True
    E   True
    Ref. (2) p. 1537

33. A True
     B True
     C False
     D False
     E False
     Ref. (2) pp. 1547–1550

34. A False
     B True
     C True
     D True
     E False
     Ref. (2) p. 2026

35. A True
     B False (exceptional)
     C True
     D True
     E False
     Ref. (2) pp. 2029–2030

36. A False (4–10%)
     B False (nicotinic acid
        deficiency)
     C True
     D True
     E False (within 48
        hours)
     Ref. (36) pp. 363–365

37. A True
     B True
     C True
     D False
     E False
     Ref. (36) pp. 400–401

38. A True
     B True
     C False
     D True
     E False
     Ref. (36) pp. 71–72

39. A False
     B True
     C True
     D False
     E False
     Ref. (19) pp. 156–157

40. A True
     B True
     C False
     D True
     E False
     Ref. (15) p. 211

41. A True
     B True
     C True
     D False
     E False
     Ref. (15) pp. 527–535

42. A True
     B False (the child
        should be given
        isoniazid-resistant
        BCG plus
        prophylactic
        isoniazid)
     C True
     D True
     E False
     Ref. (15) pp. 99–100

43. A False (type A)
     B False (rare)
     C True
     D False
     E True
     Ref. (15) pp. 338–339

44. A   False (type IV—cell
         mediated)
     B   True
     C   True
     D   False
         (type I—anaphylactic)
     E   False (type IV)
     Further examples:
     Type I: penicillin allergy,
     insect sting
     hypersensitivity
     Type II: systemic lupus
     erythematosus
     Type III: allergic
     granulomatous angiitis,
     serum sickness, lupus
     nephritis
     Type IV: allograft
     rejection, with breakdown
     one gets candidiasis,
     failure of immune
     surveillance, neoplasia
     Ref. (37) p. 20

45. A   True (methotrexate,
         azothioprine)
     B   False
     C   False
     D   True (azothioprine,
         cyclophosphamide)
     E   False
     Ref. (2) p. 1878

46. A   True
     B   True
     C   True
     D   True
     E   False (measles)
     Ref. (2) pp. 673–674

47. A   True (*Clostridium
         tetani*)
     B   True
     C   False (tetany)
     D   False (almost
         invariably alert)
     E   True
     Ref. (2) pp. 685–688

48. A   True
     B   False
     C   True
     D   True (allergic
         manifestations)
     E   False (also an allergic
         manifestation of
         tuberculosis)
     Ref. (2) pp. 701–702

49. A   True
     B   True
     C   True
     D   False
     E   False
     Ref. (2) p. 897

50. A   True
     B   True
     C   True
     D   True
     E   True
     Ref. (2) pp. 894–895

51. A   True
     B   True
     C   False
     D   False (myotonia congenita)
     E   True
     Ref. (2) p. 2041

52. A   False (usually 10 years or longer)
     B   True
     C   False (increased incidence of pulmonary tuberculosis)
     D   True
     E   False
     Ref. (2) pp. 1220–1221

53. A   True
     B   True
     C   False
     D   False
     E   True
     Ref. (3) pp. 199–200

54. A   True
     B   True
     C   False
     D   False (because they contain some galactose)
     E   False (develop over a few weeks to months)
     Ref. (2) pp. 505–506

55. A   True
     B   True
     C   False
     D   True
     E   False
     Ref. (2) pp. 1759–1761

56. A   True
     B   True (haemolytic anaemia)
     C   True
     D   True
     E   True
     Ref. (2) p. 1636

57. A   True
     B   True
     C   False
     D   True
     E   False
     Ref. (2) p. 887

58. A   False
     B   False
     C   True
     D   False (hyperparathyroidism)
     E   True
     Ref. (2) p. 102

59. A   False (blurring of vision)
     B   True
     C   False (sensitive; resistance is a normal response)
     D   True
     E   False (absent ankle jerks)
     Ref. (2) p. 108

60. A   False (always positive)
     B   True
     C   False (unlikely)
     D   False (different in value)
     E   True
     Ref. (17)

Examination 8

(Time allotted: 2½ hours)

1. **In ventricular septal defect the following are typical:**
    A   The jugular venous pressure is raised even in the absence of heart failure
    B   An apical pansystolic murmur
    C   An ejection systolic murmur may be present if pulmonary hypertension is present
    D   A Graham Steell murmur is common once pulmonary hypertension develops
    E   A fixed and widely split second heart sound

2. **Infective endocarditis is rare in:**
    A   Mixed mitral valve disease
    B   Patent ductus arteriosus
    C   Congenital bicuspid aortic stenosis
    D   Atrial septal defect
    E   Tight mitral stenosis

3. **In pulmonary atresia:**
    A   Cyanosis is present
    B   Convulsions may occur
    C   A continuous murmur is characteristic
    D   An electrocardiogram can differentiate this condition from Fallot's tetralogy
    E   Squatting may improve the symptoms

4. **Pulsus alternans:**
   A   Is characterized by an irregular rhythm
   B   Can only be diagnosed electrocardiographically
   C   Is associated with left ventricular stress
   D   May be found with atrial flutter
   E   Is typically seen in beriberi heart disease

5. ***Klebsiella* pneumonia:**
   A   Is usually mild
   B   Is commonly associated with collapse of the upper lobe
   C   Commonly produces lung abscesses
   D   Even despite adequate therapy, mortality is higher than 50%
   E   Is most commonly found in young individuals

6. **In chronic bronchitis and emphysema:**
   A   Pulmonary hypertension is common
   B   Left ventricular hypertrophy may be found
   C   The diffusion capacity is often reduced
   D   A most useful test of respiratory obstruction is the FEV_1
   E   Alpha-1-Antitrypsin deficiency may be a cause

7. **The Kveim test:**
   A   Is positive in about 80% of patients with active sarcoidosis
   B   Should be read 48–72 hours following an intra-dermal injection
   C   A false positive result may occur in Crohn's disease
   D   Corticosteroid therapy does not affect the reaction
   E   Should be done in all suspected cases to confirm the diagnosis

8. **Idiopathic pulmonary haemosiderosis:**
   A   Usually starts in the third decade
   B   Development of massive haemoptysis suggests another diagnosis
   C   Haemosiderin-laden macrophages in the sputum are diagnostic
   D   Corticosteroid therapy is contraindicated
   E   The long-term prognosis is generally good

9. **In Nelson's syndrome:**
   A   The patient may present with bitemporal hemiano-
       pia
   B   Hyperpigmentation is a very striking feature
   C   Adrenocorticotropic hormones are depressed
   D   The treatment of choice is bilateral adrenalectomy
   E   Recurrent hypoglycaemia is common

10. **Addison's disease may be associated with:**
    A   Hashimoto's thyroiditis
    B   Hyperparathyroidism
    C   Increased pigmentation
    D   Vitiligo
    E   Adrenal calcification

11. **The following statements regarding female hirsut-
    ism are true:**
    A   Coarse hair around the nipples is always abnormal
    B   Estimation of urinary 17—oxosteroids is of value
    C   Cushing's syndrome is a cause
    D   May be caused by the polycystic ovarian syndrome
    E   Phaeochromocytoma must be excluded

12. **Ankylosing spondylitis may be characterized by:**
    A   Exclusive male involvement
    B   Morning stiffness of involved joints
    C   Onset with peripheral arthropathy
    D   Severe iritis affecting vision
    E   Upper lobe fibrosing alveolitis

13. **Chondrocalcinosis may be caused by:**
    A   Hypoparathyroidism
    B   Rheumatoid arthritis
    C   Haemochromatosis
    D   Tietze's syndrome
    E   Ochronosis

14. **Hypertrophic pulmonary osteoarthropathy:**
    A   May occur in the absence of clubbing
    B   Is treated with high doses of steroids
    C   Is never unilateral
    D   Must be differentiated from pachydermoperiostitis
    E   Typically affects the distal limb long bones

15. **Cholestatic jaundice typically occurs with:**
    A Cholangiolytic hepatitis
    B Methyltestosterone therapy
    C Isoniazid therapy
    D Halothane anaesthesia
    E Biliary cirrhosis

16. **Nicotinamide deficiency produces:**
    A A high output cardiac failure
    B Dementia
    C Glossitis
    D Sensory polyneuropathy
    E Dermatitis

17. **Relatives of patients with the following disorders should be screened:**
    A Acute intermittent porphyria
    B Wilson's disease
    C Haemochromatosis
    D Gilbert's disease
    E Chlorpromazine-induced cholestatic jaundice

18. **Waldenström's macroglobulinaemia:**
    A Visual disturbances are common
    B Lymphadenopathy is rarely present
    C Polycythaemia is characteristic
    D Skeletal manifestations are frequently seen
    E Bence-Jones protein may be present in the urine

19. **The following factors assist in supporting the diagnosis of benign from malignant paraproteinaemia:**
    A Bence-Jones proteinuria
    B IgG levels of greater than 2 g/100 ml
    C Increasing levels of paraprotein
    D Normal skeletal survey
    E Asymptomatic for 2 years

20. **As regards antiepileptic therapy used in pregnancy:**
   A There is a 2–3-fold increase in incidence of birth defects if used in early pregnancy
   B Phenytoin is the drug of first choice
   C More than 90% of epileptic mothers bear normal children
   D Regular serum measurements of the drug being used are required
   E May precipitate serious haemorrhage in the first 24 hours of the neonate

21. **Nitroglycerine has the following effects:**
   A Is of significant value in Raynaud's disease only if used topically
   B Aggravates paroxysmal nocturnal dyspnoea
   C Relieves the pain of diffuse oesophageal spasm
   D May provide relief of the pain of biliary colic
   E Aggravates bronchial asthma

22. **With regards to the side-effects of D-penicillamine:**
   A Morbilliform rashes occur
   B Eosinophilia occurs
   C Loss of taste for salt results
   D Systemic lupus erythematosus–like syndrome may occur
   E Is not contraindicated in patients known to be penicillin–sensitive

23. **Thiabendazole is of value in the treatment of:**
   A *Diphyllobothrium latum*
   B *Strongyloides stercoralis*
   C *Schistosoma haematobium*
   D *Dracunculus medinensis*
   E *Wuchereria bancrofti*

24. **Cephalothin therapy:**
   A May produce a direct positive Coombs' reaction
   B Has a higher incidence of sensitivity reactions if the patient is sensitive to penicillin
   C Commonly produces renal damage
   D May reduce alkaline phosphatase
   E May produce nystagmus

25. **Doxorubicin (Adriamycin) therapy:**
    A   May be used intramuscularly
    B   Produces myelosuppression
    C   May produce cardiomyopathy
    D   Has produced excellent results in primary hepatoma
    E   Is used daily for 21 days

26. **Occlusion of the anterior spinal artery:**
    A   Produces loss of joint position sense
    B   May produce spastic paraparesis
    C   Usually produces retention of urine and of faeces
    D   Prognosis is good even in severe cases
    E   May occur in following a massive gastrointestinal haemorrhage

27. **Migraine is characterized by the following:**
    A   Cannot be diagnosed in the absence of prodromal symptoms
    B   Fortification spectra
    C   Homonymous hemianopia
    D   Papilloedema
    E   Common occurrence of auditory hallucinations

28. **Progressive spinal muscular atrophy of infancy may present with:**
    A   Severe generalized weakness
    B   Fasciculations seen in the tongue
    C   Loss of spinothalamic tract function
    D   Spontaneous fibrillation on electromyography
    E   Raised cerebrospinal fluid protein

29. **Complications of meningococcal meningitis include:**
    A   Hydrocephalus
    B   Paraparesis
    C   Cortical blindness
    D   Deafness
    E   Peripheral neuropathy

30. **Pulmonary fibrosis:**
   A   May follow staphylococcal pneumonia
   B   Is associated with cough and expectoration
   C   May be produced by high concentration asbestos exposure
   D   May produce bronchial breathing if massive pulmonary fibrosis is present
   E   Is excluded if crepitations are absent

31. **Dysarthria occurs with:**
   A   General paralysis of the insane
   B   Friedreich's ataxia
   C   Motor neurone disease
   D   Charcot–Marie–Tooth disease
   E   Moebius' syndrome

32. **Dysphagia may be produced by:**
   A   Oesophageal varices
   B   Severe mitral stenosis
   C   Motor neurone disease
   D   Ménétrièr's disease
   E   Severe thyrotoxicosis

33. **Systemic sclerosis may affect gastrointestinal tract as follows:**
   A   Perforation of the colon
   B   Increased incidence of carcinoma of the oesophagus
   C   Higher association with regional ileitis
   D   Pseudodiverticuli on radiology
   E   Ileus

34. **In pyloric stenosis of infancy:**
   A   Inheritance is autosomal dominant
   B   Vomiting usually begins in the 1st week
   C   The vomit is frequently bile-stained
   D   An abdominal tumour is almost always palpable
   E   Complications commonly develop in adulthood

35. **The following foods must be avoided in coeliac disease (gluten enteropathy):**
   A   Cheese
   B   Corn flakes
   C   Rye cereals
   D   Beer
   E   Bread

36. **Unconjugated hyperbilirubinaemia is typical of:**
   A   Dubin–Johnson syndrome
   B   Hereditary spherocytosis
   C   Rotor's syndrome
   D   Gilbert's disease
   E   Biliary atresia

37. **Familial hepatic diseases associated with cirrhosis include:**
   A   Galactosaemia
   B   Osler–Weber–Rendu syndrome
   C   Cystinosis
   D   Marfan's syndrome
   E   Wilson's disease

38. **Complications of smallpox vaccination include:**
   A   Erythema nodosum
   B   Erythema multiforme
   C   Encephalitis 2 days following vaccination
   D   Haemolytic anaemia
   E   Interstitial nephritis

39. **Febrile convulsions:**
   A   Never present with a focal onset
   B   May be associated with a positive family history of febrile convulsions
   C   May show a normal interictal electroencephalogram
   D   Have a high recurrence rate
   E   Never produce brain damage

40. **Causes of mental retardation include:**
    A   Severe malnutrition
    B   Poliomyelitis
    C   Cri-du-chat syndrome
    D   Cytomegalic inclusion disease
    E   Syringomyelia

41. **Psychosis in children is suggested by:**
    A   Absence of speech
    B   Intense outbursts of temper
    C   Recurrence of bedwetting following a period of control
    D   Feelings of depersonalization
    E   Sudden onset of stuttering

42. **In differentiating psychoneurosis from psychosis:**
    A   The neurotic characteristically denies the existence of reality
    B   Inner experiences severely upset external behaviour in neurosis
    C   True delusions may occur in neurosis
    D   Associations are unimpaired in neurosis
    E   The ego remains sound in the neurotic

43. **In autosomal dominant inheritance:**
    A   There is a 25% risk of involvement in the siblings
    B   The disease is usually not so serious as a recessively inherited one
    C   There are affected individuals in several generations
    D   Normal parents are carriers
    E   The rarer the trait the greater the incidence of consanguinity in the family

44. **The following are true regarding sympathetic ophthalmia:**
   A   It may follow surgery for cataract
   B   Presence of photophobia excludes the diagnosis
   C   Pathologically there is diffuse granulomatous uveitis
   D   It only follows years after initial injury
   E   If enucleation is performed within 10 days after injury the condition can almost invariably be averted

45. **Plague:**
   A   May be acquired by droplet infection in man
   B   Usually does not produce any pyrexia
   C   Produces painful and swollen lymph glands enlargement
   D   Produces characteristic circinate rashes
   E   Responds to penicillin therapy in large doses

46. **In amoebic dysentery:**
   A   Symptoms may resemble those of a duodenal ulcer
   B   Periods of alternating diarrhoea and constipation suggest an associated underlying carcinoma
   C   The motions are not offensive-smelling
   D   Hepatic amoebiasis is a rare complication
   E   Metronidazole is the treatment of first choice

47. *Toxocara canis:*
   A   Produces severe pruritis *in ano*
   B   Produces hepatosplenomegaly
   C   May produce asthma
   D   Larval forms respond to diethylcarbamazine therapy
   E   Produces chronic diarrhoea in children

48. **Sulphonamide therapy may produce:**
   A   Bazin's disease
   B   Cyanosis
   C   Morphoea
   D   Photosensitivity with topical use
   E   Haematuria

49. **Lymphogranuloma venereum:**
   A   Is common in temperate climates
   B   Characteristically produces a normal erythrocyte sedimentation rate
   C   Is due to a Bedsonia organism
   D   Usually produces a herpetiform primary lesion
   E   May produce a non-gonococcal urethritis

50. **Retroperitoneal fibrosis is associated with:**
   A   Extensive ureteric obstruction
   B   Bile duct obstruction
   C   Hashimoto's thyroiditis
   D   Peyronie's disease of the penis
   E   Busulphan therapy

51. **Laboratory features of early nephrotic syndrome include:**
   A   Albumin less than 2.5 g/100 ml
   B   Decreased fibrinogen
   C   Elevated alpha-2-globulin
   D   Elevated serum creatinine
   E   Decreased erythrocyte sedimentation rate

52. **A large kidney is produced by:**
   A   Post-obstructive uropathy
   B   Polycystic renal disease
   C   Chronic glomerulonephritis
   D   Renal amyloidosis
   E   Hypertrophy following contralateral nephrectomy

53. **Cicatricial alopecia is typically caused by:**
   A   X-ray therapy or ringworm of the scalp
   B   Alopecia areata
   C   Discoid lupus erythematosus
   D   Postpartum state
   E   Heparin therapy

54. **Infectious mononucleosis characteristically presents with:**
   A   Periorbital swelling
   B   Generalized lymphadenopathy
   C   Jaundice in the majority of patients
   D   Palatal petechiae
   E   Pruritis

55. **In polycythaemia rubra vera:**
   A   Transient visual disturbances occur
   B   Tendency to thrombosis only affects the veins
   C   The Budd–Chiari syndrome may result
   D   Gastrointestinal bleeding occurs
   E   Gout is very rare

56. **The following are true about chronic lymphocytic lymphoma:**
   A   Previous irradiation is an aetiological factor
   B   In half the cases it starts under the age of 30 years
   C   Splenic enlargement produces pain
   D   A Coombs' negative haemolytic anaemia may be present
   E   Hypogammaglobulinaemia is frequently present

57. **Beta thalassaemia is characterized by:**
   A   Hepatosplenomegaly
   B   Overgrowth of maxillary regions of the face
   C   A lower incidence of infections
   D   A normal reticulocyte count
   E   Characteristic changes on x-ray of the skull

58. **Cardiac output is increased by:**
   A   Sleep
   B   Tachyarrhythmias of a rate greater than 200/minute
   C   Eating
   D   Moderate changes in environment
   E   Sitting up from a lying position

59. **The following statements are true:**

A The 1st part of the duodenum is overlapped by the liver and gall bladder

B The 2nd part of the duodenum is crossed by the pancreas

C The ampulla of Vater is situated on the 3rd part of the duodenum

D The superior pancreaticoduodenal artery arises from the superior mesenteric artery

E The right kidney lies directly behind the 2nd part of the duodenum

60. **The following statements are true:**

A The Pearsonian measure of skewness is based upon the sum of the arithmetic mean and the mode

B In a symmetrical distribution the mean, median and the mode are all equal

C The term census refers to a full count of the specific population

D The larger the sample the greater will be the standard error

E The observed result with a probability of 0.02 is more significant than with a probability of 0.05

OFFICIAL
USE ONLY

SURNAME	INITIALS
JOSHI	P

CANDIDATE NUMBER

THOU. 0 1 2 3 4 5 6 7 8 9

HUND. 0 1 2 3 4 5 6 7 8 9

4 7 5 6

TENS 0 1 2 3 4 5 6 7 8 9

UNITS 0 1 2 3 4 5 6 7 8 9

PAGE No.
1

T means TRUE F means FALSE D means DO NOT KNOW

	1A	1B	1C	1D	1E		2A	2B	2C	2D	2E
1	T F D	T F D	T F D	T F D	T F D	2	T F D	T F D	T F D	T F D	T F D

	3A	3B	3C	3D	3E		4A	4B	4C	4D	4E
3	T F D	T F D	T F D	T F D	T F D	4	T F D	T F D	T F D	T F D	T F D

	5A	5B	5C	5D	5E		6A	6B	6C	6D	6E
5	T F D	T F D	T F D	T F D	T F D	6	T F D	T F D	T F D	T F D	T F D

	7A	7B	7C	7D	7E		8A	8B	8C	8D	8E
7	T F D	T F D	T F D	T F D	T F D	8	T F D	T F D	T F D	T F D	T F D

	9A	9B	9C	9D	9E		10A	10B	10C	10D	10E
9	T F D	T F D	T F D	T F D	T F D	10	T F D	T F D	T F D	T F D	T F D

	11A	11B	11C	11D	11E		12A	12B	12C	12D	12E
11	T F D	T F D	T F D	T F D	T F D	12	T F D	T F D	T F D	T F D	T F D

	13A	13B	13C	13D	13E		14A	14B	14C	14D	14E
13	T F D	T F D	T F D	T F D	T F D	14	T F D	T F D	T F D	T F D	T F D

	15A	15B	15C	15D	15E		16A	16B	16C	16D	16E
15	T F D	T F D	T F D	T F D	T F D	16	T F D	T F D	T F D	T F D	T F D

	17A	17B	17C	17D	17E		18A	18B	18C	18D	18E
17	T F D	T F D	T F D	T F D	T F D	18	T F D	T F D	T F D	T F D	T F D

	19A	19B	19C	19D	19E		20A	20B	20C	20D	20E
19	T F D	T F D	T F D	T F D	T F D	20	T F D	T F D	T F D	T F D	T F D

	21A	21B	21C	21D	21E		22A	22B	22C	22D	22E
21	T F D	T F D	T F D	T F D	T F D	22	T F D	T F D	T F D	T F D	T F D

	23A	23B	23D	23C	23E		24A	24B	24C	24D	24E
23	T F D	T F D	T F D	T F D	T F D	24	T F D	T F D	T F D	T F D	T F D

	25A	25B	25C	25D	25E		26A	26B	26C	26D	26E
25	T F D	T F D	T F D	T F D	T F D	26	T F D	T F D	T F D	T F D	T F D

	27A	27B	27C	27D	27E		28A	28B	28C	28D	28E
27	T F D	T F D	T F D	T F D	T F D	28	T F D	T F D	T F D	T F D	T F D

	29A	29B	29C	29D	29E		30A	30B	30C	30D	30E
29	T F D	T F D	T F D	T F D	T F D	30	T F D	T F D	T F D	T F D	T F D

168

SURNAME	INITIALS
JOSHI	P

CANDIDATE NUMBER

THOU. 0 1 2 3 4 5 6 7 8 9

HUND. 0 1 2 3 4 5 6 7 8 9

4 7 5 6

TENS 0 1 2 3 4 5 6 7 8 9

UNITS 0 1 2 3 4 5 6 7 8 9

PAGE No.
1

T means TRUE F means FALSE D means DO NOT KNOW

	31A	31B	31C	31D	31E		32A	32B	32C	32D	32E
31	T F D	T F D	T F D	T F D	T F D	32	T F D	T F D	T F D	T F D	T F D

	33A	33B	33C	33D	33E		34A	34B	34C	34D	34E
33	T F D	T F D	T F D	T F D	T F D	34	T F D	T F D	T F D	T F D	T F D

	35A	35B	35C	35D	35E		36A	36B	36C	36D	36E
35	T F D	T F D	T F D	T F D	T F D	36	T F D	T F D	T F D	T F D	T F D

	37A	37B	37C	37D	37E		38A	38B	38C	38D	38E
37	T F D	T F D	T F D	T F D	T F D	38	T F D	T F D	T F D	T F D	T F D

	39A	39B	39C	39D	39E		40A	40B	40C	40D	40E
39	T F D	T F D	T F D	T F D	T F D	40	T F D	T F D	T F D	T F D	T F D

	41A	41B	41C	41D	41E		42A	42B	42C	43D	43E
41	T F D	T F D	T F D	T F D	T F D	42	T F D	T F D	T F D	T F D	T F D

	43A	43B	43C	43D	43E		44A	44B	44C	44D	44E
43	T F D	T F D	T F D	T F D	T F D	44	T F D	T F D	T F D	T F D	T F D

	45A	45B	45C	45D	45E		46A	46B	46C	46D	46E
45	T F D	T F D	T F D	T F D	T F D	46	T F D	T F D	T F D	T F D	T F D

	47A	47B	47C	47D	47E		48A	48B	48C	48D	48E
47	T F D	T F D	T F D	T F D	T F D	48	T F D	T F D	T F D	T F D	T F D

	49A	49B	49C	49D	49E		50A	50B	50C	50D	50E
49	T F D	T F D	T F D	T F D	T F D	50	T F D	T F D	T F D	T F D	T F D

	51A	51B	51C	51D	51E		52A	52B	52C	52D	52E
51	T F D	T F D	T F D	T F D	T F D	52	T F D	T F D	T F D	T F D	T F D

	53A	53B	53C	53D	53E		54A	54B	54C	54D	54E
53	T F D	T F D	T F D	T F D	T F D	54	T F D	T F D	T F D	T F D	T F D

	55A	55B	55C	55D	55E		56A	56B	56C	56D	56E
55	T F D	T F D	T F D	T F D	T F D	56	T F D	T F D	T F D	T F D	T F D

	57A	57B	57C	57D	57E		58A	58B	58C	58D	58E
57	T F D	T F D	T F D	T F D	T F D	58	T F D	T F D	T F D	T F D	T F D

	59A	59B	59C	59D	59E		60A	60B	60C	60D	60E
59	T F D	T F D	T F D	T F D	T F D	60	T F D	T F D	T F D	T F D	T F D

Answers to Examination 8
(For complete References see Chapter 3)

1.   A   False (normal)
     B   False (typically in the
           3rd–4th left
           intercostal space)
     C   True
     D   False
     E   False
     Ref. (*10*) pp. 268–285

2.   A   False
     B   False
     C   False
     D   True
     E   True
     Ref. (*10*) pp. 366, 411, 418,
   433, 444

3.   A   True
     B   True
     C   True (because of
           proximal
           bronchopulmonary
           anastomosis)
     D   False
     E   True
     Ref. (*10*) p. 352

4.   A   False (regular)
     B   False
     C   True
     D   True
     E   False
     Ref. (*10*) p. 30

5.   A   False (severe)
     B   False (bulging of the
           fissure occurs
           because of an intense
           inflammatory
           exudate)
     C   True
     D   False
     E   False
     Ref. (*40*) pp. 137–138

6.   A   True (because of
           hypoxia)
     B   True (in 25–60% of
           cases)
     C   True
     D   True
     E   True
     Ref. (*40*) pp. 330–335

7.   A   True
     B   False (lesion should
           be biopsied 4–6
           weeks later)
     C   True
     D   False
     E   False
     Ref. (*9*) p. 224

8. A   False (in childhood)
    B   False
    C   False (may occur in any disease associated with lung haemorrhage)
    D   False (it may produce temporary remissions)
    E   False (variable—but usually die within 5 years)
    Ref. (*9*) p. 263
          (*8*) p. 915

9. A   True (a feature of a pituitary tumour)
    B   True (because increased levels of melanocyte stimulating hormone)
    C   False
    D   False
    E   False
    Ref. (*9*) pp. 14, 39

10. A   True
    B   False (hypoparathyroidism)
    C   True
    D   True
    E   True (suggests tuberculosis)
    Ref. (*9*) pp. 43–44

11. A   False
    B   True (because of androgen secretion)
    C   True
    D   True
    E   False
    Ref. (*9*) pp. 175–178

12. A   False
    B   True (often)
    C   True (10%)
    D   False (rarely more than slight ocular discomfort)
    E   True
    Ref. (*1*) pp. 107–111

13. A   False (hyperparathyroidism)
    B   False
    C   True
    D   False
    E   True
    Ref. (*1*) pp. 138–139

14. A   False
    B   False
    C   False (an arteriovenous aneurysm should be suspected)
    D   True
    E   True
    Ref. (*1*) pp. 152–153

15. A   True
    B   True
    C   False
    D   False
    E   True
    Ref. (*42*) p. 269

16. A   False (thiamine deficiency—beri beri)
    B   True
    C   True
    D   False
    E   True
    Ref. (*42*) p. 357

17. A   True
     B   True
     C   True
     D   False
     E   False
     Also true for the
     following:
     Cholinesterase
     abnormalities
     Glucose-6-phosphate
     dehydrogenase deficiency
     Porphyria variegata
     Cystinuria
     Ref. (42) pp. 334–335

18. A   True
     B   False (often)
     C   False (anaemia)
     D   False (not seen)
     E   True (10%)
     Ref. (42) p. 243

19. A   False (malignant)
     B   False (malignant)
     C   False (malignant)
     D   True
     E   True
     Ref. (42) pp. 244–245

20. A   True
     B   False
     C   True
     D   False
     E   True
     Ref. (6) p. 471

21. A   True
     B   False (provides
           dramatic relief)
     C   True
     D   True
     E   False (may improve
           it)
     Ref. (6) pp. 825–828

22. A   True (also pruritic,
           and urticarial rashes)
     B   True
     C   True (also for sweet
           taste)
     D   True
     E   False
     Indications for
     D-penicillamine include:
     Wilson's disease
     Lead poisoning
     Cystinuria
     Primary biliary cirrhosis
     Scleroderma, etc
     Ref. (6) pp. 1627–1628

23. A   False (niclosamide,
           dichlorophen)
     B   True
     C   False (niridazole,
           stibophen,
           hycanthone,
           antimonials,
           oxamniquine)
     D   True
     E   False
           (diethylcarbamazine)
     Ref. (6) p. 1027

24. A   True (40% when
           high doses are used)
     B   True
     C   False (rarely)
     D   False (produces a
           transient increase)
     E   True
     Ref. (6) pp. 1153–1154

25. A   False (intravenously)
     B   True
     C   True
     D   False
     E   False (single
           intravenous dose
           every 21 days)
     Ref. (6) pp. 1291–1293

26. A   False
    B   True
    C   True
    D   False
    E   True
    Ref. (*43*) pp. 784–785

27. A   False
    B   True
    C   True
    D   False
    E   False (rare)
    Ref. (*43*) pp. 302–305

28. A   True
    B   True
    C   False
    D   True
    E   False
    Ref. (*43*) pp. 705–706

29. A   True
    B   True
    C   False
    D   True
    E   False
    Ref. (*43*) pp. 415–416

30. A   True
    B   False (unless
         associated with or
         complicated by
         infection or
         bronchiectasis)
    C   True
    D   True
    E   False
    Ref. (*59*) pp. 1469–1470,
    1894

31. A   True
    B   True
    C   True
    D   False
    E   True (bilateral lower
         motor neurone type
         facial paralysis)
    Ref. (*22*) pp. 324, 349,
    352, 355, 384, 391

32. A   False (produces
         severe
         haematemesis)
    B   True (aneurysmal
         left atrium
         compresses the
         oesophagus)
    C   True (bulbar or
         pseudobulbar palsy)
    D   False
    E   True (compression
         by the goitre may
         occur)
    Ref. (*22*) pp. 201, 282,
    297, 349, 352, 353, 355,
    384, 391, 435

33. A   True
    B   False
    C   False
    D   True
    E   True
    Ref. (*28k*) p. 32

34. A   False (not an
         inherited disorder)
    B   False (2–4 weeks
         later)
    C   False (may suggest
         an annular pancreas)
    D   True
    E   False
    Ref. (*25*) pp. 510–511

35.	A	False	40.	A	True
	B	False		B	False
	C	True		C	True
	D	True		D	True
	E	True		E	False
	Ref. (25) p. 539			Ref. (25) pp. 186–188	

36.	A	False (conjugated)	41.	A	True
	B	True		B	True
	C	False		C	False
	D	True		D	True
	E	False		E	False
	Ref. (25) pp. 554–555			Ref. (25) pp. 712–717	

37.	A	True	42.	A	False
	B	True		B	False
	C	False		C	False
	D	False		D	True
	E	True		E	True
	Ref. (25) p. 562			Ref. (19) pp. 459–460	

38.	A	False	43.	A	False (50%)
	B	True		B	True
	C	False (10–13 days later)		C	True
	D	True (unusual)		D	False
	E	False		E	False
				Ref. (25) p. 1007	

Also rarely seen are the following:
Arthritis
Osteomyelitis
Pericarditis
Myocarditis
Ref. (25) p. 821

			44.	A	True
				B	False
				C	True
				D	False (10 days to years later)
39.	A	False (rarely they do)		E	True
	B	True (in 40%)		Ref. (23) pp. 116–117	
	C	False			
	D	True	45.	A	True
	E	False (may if prolonged)		B	False
	Ref. (25) pp. 641–642			C	True
				D	False
				E	False (streptomycin or tetracyclines)
				Ref. (52) pp. 749–750	

46. A True
    B False (frequently present)
    C False (offensive stools)
    D False (common)
    E True
    Ref. (52) pp. 773–775

47. A False
    B True
    C True
    D True
    E False
    Ref. (52) p. 800

48. A False
    B True (due to methaemoglobin-aemia)
    C False
    D True
    E True
    Ref. (52) p. 42

49. A False
    B False
    C True
    D True
    E True
    Ref. (8) pp. 121–122

50. A False (localized ureteric obstruction occurs)
    B True (from periductal fibrosis)
    C False (Riedl's thyroiditis)
    D True
    E False
    Ref. (5) pp. 99–102

51. A True
    B False (increased)
    C True
    D False (normal)
    E False (often increased)
    Ref. (5) pp. 63–64

52. A True
    B True
    C False (small)
    D True
    E True
    Ref. (5) pp. 193–194

53. A True
    B False
    C True
    D False
    E False
    Ref. (8) pp. 1242–1245

54. A True
    B True
    C False (15%)
    D True
    E False
    Ref. (8) p. 1174

55. A True
    B False (also affects the arteries)
    C True
    D True
    E False
    Ref. (8) pp. 1189–1191

56. A   False (acute and
         chronic myeloid
         leukaemia)
     B   False
     C   False
     D   True (also a
         Coombs' positive
         haemolytic anaemia)
     E   True (in 60%)
     Ref. (8) p. 1199

57. A   True
     B   True
     C   False (higher
         incidence)
     D   False
     E   True
     Ref. (8) pp. 1160–1161

58. A   False (no change)
     B   False (decreased)
     C   True (increased by
         up to 30%)
     D   False
     E   False (decreases by
         20–30%)
     Ref. (21)

59. A   True
     B   False
     C   False
     D   False (it arises from
         the gastroduodenal
         artery)
     E   True
     Ref. (14) pp. 88–91

60. A   False (it is based on
         the difference
         between the
         arithmetic mean and
         the mode)
     B   True
     C   True
     D   False (the smaller
         will be the standard
         error)
     E   True
     Ref. (17)

Examination 9
(Time allotted: 2½ hours)

1. **Delayed hypersensitivity is impaired in:**
   A   Wiscott–Aldrich syndrome
   B   Hereditary haemorrhagic telengiectasia
   C   Sarcoidosis
   D   DiGeorge syndrome
   E   Chronic giardiasis

2. **Acute rheumatic fever is frequently associated with the following electrocardiographic changes:**
   A   Shortened P–R interval
   B   Non-paroxysmal atrioventricular nodal tachycardia
   C   3rd degree atrioventricular block
   D   Prolonged Q–T interval
   E   Tall symmetrical T waves in the precordial leads

3. **The following statements are true regarding aortic incompetence:**
   A   The early diastolic murmur appearing during acute rheumatic valvulitis is usually transient
   B   Angina pectoris is more commonly present than in aortic stenosis
   C   Increasing degrees of incompetence regularly produce a louder murmur
   D   A loud 1st heart sound differentiates an Austin Flint murmur from organic mitral stenosis
   E   A presystolic murmur (accentuation) may occur even without associated mitral stenosis

4. **In patients with tetralogy of Fallot:**
   A   Sudden cyanotic attacks are characteristic
   B   The murmur is produced by flow across the ventricular septal defect
   C   Clubbing is typically found only in the fingers and not the toes
   D   Repeated cardiac failure is common
   E   A dominant 'a' wave on the jugular venous pressure is common

5. **Blood cholesterol may be reduced in coronary atherosclerosis by the following drugs:**
   A   Saccharine
   B   Nicotinic acid
   C   Clofibrate (Atromid S)
   D   Sulphinpyrazone
   E   Thyroxine

6. **The following statements are true:**
   A   The left coronary artery divides into the anterior descending and circumflex branches
   B   The circumflex branch runs in the interventricular groove
   C   The anterior walls of the left and right ventricles are supplied by the right coronary artery
   D   The diagonal branch supplies the anterolateral aspect of the left ventricle
   E   In 90% of subjects the left coronary artery is the dominant artery

7. **Eye involvement in arthritic patients includes:**
   A   Cytoid bodies in systemic lupus erythematosus
   B   Episcleritis in Behçet's disease
   C   Chorioretinitis in Still's disease
   D   Hypopyon in Behçet's disease
   E   Iridocyclitis in ankylosing spondylitis

8. **Severe aspirin poisoning may produce:**
   A   Hypocalcaemia
   B   Hypoglycaemia
   C   Hyperprothrombinaemia
   D   Ototoxicity
   E   Bone marrow depression

9. **Familial Mediterranean fever is characterized by:**
   A   Autosomal dominant inheritance
   B   Abdominal pain
   C   Large-joint polyarthritis
   D   Pathognomonic synovial membrane biopsy
   E   Amyloidosis of the perireticulin distribution

10. **In polymyalgia rheumatica:**
    A   Onset is in the mid-forties
    B   Early morning joint stiffness is typical
    C   Females are more commonly affected than males
    D   The erythrocyte sedimentation rate is typically normal
    E   Electromyographic changes are characteristically abnormal

11. **Serum bicarbonate = 30 mmol/litre (30 mEq/litre), Pa_{CO_2} = 52 mmHg, pH = 7.2. The following are possible causes:**
    A   Mild asthma
    B   Diabetic ketoacidosis
    C   Barbiturate poisoning
    D   Prolonged vomiting
    E   Chronic bronchitis

12. **Mycoplasma infections:**
    A   Commonly produce a pneumonia
    B   May be accompanied by otitis media
    C   May produce the Stevens–Johnson syndrome
    D   Respond satisfactorily to high dose sulphonamide therapy
    E   May produce a haemolytic anaemia

13. **Bilateral pleural effusions are seen in:**
    A   Pleural mesothelioma
    B   Systemic lupus erythematosus
    C   Miliary tuberculosis
    D   Lymphangitis carcinomatosa
    E   Sarcoidosis

14. **In a patient with breathlessness both the FEV_1 and FVC are reduced, with a FEV_1/FVC ratio of 82%. The differential diagnosis would include:**
    A   Acute asthma
    B   Fibrosing alveolitis
    C   Pleural effusion
    D   Ankylosing spondylitis
    E   Chronic bronchitis

15. **Killed organisms are used for immunization in the following:**
    A   Typhoid
    B   Poliomyelitis (Salk) vaccine
    C   Measles
    D   Rubella
    E   Bacille–Calmette–Guérin (BCG)

16. **Classic features of disseminated sclerosis include:**
    A   Paraesthesiae
    B   Retrobulbar neuritis
    C   Impairment of position and vibration senses
    D   Diplopia
    E   Unremitting progression

17. **In petit mal epilepsy:**
    A   Causative cerebral tumours may be found
    B   Breath-holding spells occur
    C   Characteristic electroencephalographic changes are seen
    D   Grand mal seizures may occur if the disorder continues into adulthood
    E   Treatment is of little value

18. **Fasciculations occur in:**
   A   Amyotrophic lateral sclerosis
   B   Poliomyelitis
   C   Spinal muscular atrophy
   D   Charcot–Marie–Tooth disease
   E   Pseudohypertrophic muscular dystrophy

19. **The following entrapment neuropathies are well described:**
   A   Carpal tunnel syndrome affecting the median nerve
   B   Tic douloureux affecting the trigeminal nerve
   C   Pronator syndrome affecting the posterior interosseus nerve
   D   Morton's metatarsalgia affecting the plantar nerve
   E   Meralgia paraesthetica affecting the lateral femoral cutaneous nerve

20. **Marburg virus disease is characterized clinically by:**
   A   Marked lumbar myalgia
   B   Erythematous rash on the 5th day
   C   Gastrointestinal haemorrhage
   D   Severe tachycardia
   E   Generalized lymphadenopathy as a constant feature

21. **Blackwater fever:**
   A   May occur with quartan malaria
   B   Produces acute tubular necrosis
   C   Only occurs in patients given antimalarials
   D   Produces an over 80% mortality
   E   Usually has an absence of a parasitaemia

22. **Cryptococcal infections produce:**
   A   Diplopia
   B   Jacksonian convulsions
   C   Pulmonary cavitation
   D   Pleural effusions commonly
   E   Typical calcified hilar adenopathy

23. **The following tests are useful in differentiating non-tropical sprue from pancreatic insufficiency:**
   A   Urinary indican
   B   D-xylose test
   C   Schilling test
   D   Serum albumin
   E   Serum cholesterol

24. **Acquired megacolon may occur in:**
   A   Chagas' disease
   B   Amyloidosis
   C   Hypothermia
   D   Carcinoid syndrome
   E   Spinal cord injury

25. **Irritable colon syndrome classically presents with:**
   A   Lower abdominal pain aggravated by defaecation
   B   Alternating constipation and diarrhoea
   C   Passage of small-calibre stools
   D   Dysentery
   E   Recurrent episodes of vomiting

26. **Drug-induced colitis:**
   A   May be produced by Ampicillin
   B   Characteristically produces bloody diarrhoea
   C   Produces fever
   D   Should be treated with corticosteroids in most cases
   E   May follow the use of cholestyramine

27. **The following conditions are associated with skin involvement and a higher incidence of internal malignancy:**
   A   Neurofibromatosis
   B   Gardner's syndrome
   C   Peutz–Jegher's syndrome
   D   Tuberous sclerosis
   E   Fanconi's anaemia

28. **Effects of atropine include:**
   A Slight cardiac slowing in a dose of 0.5 mg
   B Meiosis
   C Blurring of vision
   D Urinary incontinence
   E Ataxia

29. **Cyproheptadine (Periactin):**
   A May be used as an antipruritic agent
   B Is of value in the postgastrectomy dumping syndrome
   C Is used for the intestinal hypermotility of carcinoid syndrome
   D Quite commonly causes weight loss in children
   E May be used as an appetite suppressant

30. **Quinidine:**
   A Is of little value in the treatment of atrial fibrillation
   B Produces prolongation of the Q–T interval on electrocardiogram
   C May produce cinchonism
   D May produce transient ventricular tachycardia
   E Is contraindicated in the treatment of digitalis toxicity

31. **Untoward effects of oxygen inhalation include:**
   A Pulmonary atelectasis
   B Hepatic fibrosis
   C Retrolental fibroplasia
   D Acute renal failure
   E Myocardial depression

32. **Bence–Jones proteins:**
   A Produce a positive urinary test with albustix
   B Increase in amount in the urine with impairment of renal function
   C Are rarely found in benign monoclonal gammopathy
   D If severe, result in hypoproteinaemia
   E Are light chain proteins

33. **Drug-induced systemic lupus erythematosus:**
   A   Frequently produces renal involvement
   B   Produces arthritis
   C   May require corticosteroid therapy
   D   Is produced by pyrazinamide
   E   Produces pericarditis

34. **Hypothyroidism may be produced:**
   A   Following radio-iodine therapy
   B   By para-aminosalicylic acid therapy
   C   By iodine overdosage
   D   By indomethacin therapy
   E   By Hashimoto's disease

35. **Excessive androgen production produces:**
   A   Temporal balding
   B   Menorrhagia
   C   Acne
   D   Loss of libido
   E   Hirsutism

36. **Non-diabetic glycosuria may be found in:**
   A   Fanconi's syndrome
   B   Heavy metal poisoning
   C   Furosemide therapy
   D   Brain tumours
   E   Potassium deficiency

37. **Radio-opaque renal stones are seen with:**
   A   Calcium oxalate stones
   B   Xanthine stones
   C   Uric acid stones
   D   Cystine stones
   E   Magnesium-ammonium-phosphate stones

38. **Jaundice and acute renal failure occur in:**
   A   *Amanita phalloides* poisoning
   B   Gram-negative septicaemias
   C   Weil's disease
   D   Polycystic kidneys
   E   Salicylate poisoning

39. **A serum calcium level of 12 mg% (3.0 mmol/litre) is compatible with:**
   A   Acute alcoholic pancreatitis
   B   Myelomatosis
   C   Hypothyroidism
   D   Renal tubular acidosis
   E   sarcoidosis

40. **Hyperuricaemia is associated with:**
   A   Reticuloses
   B   Haemolytic states
   C   Pre-eclampsia
   D   Acute alcoholic overdosage
   E   Hypoparathyroidism

41. **Autosomal dominant inheritance is present in:**
   A   Ehlers–Danlos syndrome
   B   Homocystinuria
   C   Hereditary spherocytosis
   D   Galactosaemia
   E   Marfan's syndrome

42. **Retinitis pigmentosa:**
   A   May be causally related to systemic lupus erythematosus
   B   Produces night blindness
   C   May be associated with glaucoma
   D   Is associated with the Laurence–Moon–Biedl syndrome
   E   The involvement is always bilateral

43. **Regarding the chi-square test:**
   A   It is the measure of the overall difference between the observed and expected frequencies
   B   The greater the value of chi-square the less likely it is to be significant
   C   It is always less than zero
   D   The number of degrees of freedom is the number of independent comparisons involved in any chi-square test
   E   The null hypothesis has to be applied

44. **Clubbing of the nails may be found in:**
   A   Chronic meningococcal meningitis
   B   Rheumatoid arthritis
   C   Tetralogy of Fallot
   D   Schistosomiasis
   E   Iatrogenic myxoedema

45. **Impetigo:**
   A   Is usually due to a staphylococcal infection
   B   Produces blistering
   C   May be complicated by toxic epidermal necrolysis
   D   Usually affects unexposed areas of the body
   E   Is rarely contagious

46. **Reiter's disease:**
   A   Usually produces a monoarthritis
   B   Produces mucocutaneous lesions
   C   Usually presents with a normal erythrocyte sedimentation rate
   D   Produces eye lesions which commonly appear months to years after onset of the illness
   E   May produce sacroiliitis

47. **In kala-azar (visceral leishmaniasis):**
   A   Infection is always followed by overt disease
   B   Gross splenomegaly occurs
   C   Jaundice occurs commonly
   D   Hyperpigmentation occurs
   E   Mortality is unusual even without treatment

48. **Burkitt's lymphoma:**
   A   May be causally related to the Ebstein–Barr virus
   B   May present with paraplegia
   C   Has a poor prognosis regardless of treatment
   D   May produce a malignant meningitis
   E   Occurs chiefly in adults

49. **The following features are compatible with a diagnosis of chronic lymphocytic leukaemia:**
   A   Peripheral lymphocyte count of 5400/mm^3
   B   Platelet count of 750 000/mm^3
   C   Enlarged tender spleen
   D   Acute blastic transformation
   E   Positive direct antiglobulin (Coombs') test

50. **Bleeding due to a platelet defect as opposed to a coagulation defect is suggested by:**
   A   Haemarthrosis
   B   Bleeding from superficial scratches
   C   Immediate profuse bleeding following a tooth extraction
   D   Mucosal bleeding
   E   Menorrhagia

51. **In classic haemophilia:**
   A   Inheritance is autosomal recessive
   B   All the sons of an affected man will be affected
   C   50% of the daughters of a transmitter female will be transmitters
   D   Haematuria may occur
   E   Spontaneous haemorrhage in the brain is common

52. **Psychiatric disorders are associated with the following underlying systemic disorders:**
   A   Islet-cell tumour of the pancreas
   B   Gout
   C   Pernicious anaemia
   D   Reiter's disease
   E   Acute cholecystitis

53. **In catatonic schizophrenia:**
   A   Phases of excitement characteristically occur
   B   Occurrence is typically between the ages of 40–60 years
   C   Automatism is a prominent feature
   D   Urinary incontinence is common
   E   The patient may suddenly become aggressive

54. **In Huntington's chorea:**
    A   Onset is usually acute
    B   Hallucinations may occur
    C   Extreme dementia may occur
    D   Choreiform movements usually first affect the lower extremities
    E   Tendon reflexes are increased

55. **In grand mal epilepsy:**
    A   Sudden cessation of phenobarbital therapy may produce status epilepticus
    B   Mesantoin therapy may be safely combined with Tridione therapy
    C   Acetazolamide (Diamox) is of value in the treatment
    D   Phenothiazine therapy is contraindicated
    E   Imipramine may be safely used if associated depression is present

56. **The following congenital heart diseases produce central cyanosis:**
    A   Total anomalous pulmonary venous drainage
    B   Pulmonary stenosis
    C   Severe aortic stenosis
    D   Tricuspid atresia
    E   Ebstein's anomaly

57. **Features of infantile rickets include:**
    A   Muscular hypertonia
    B   Head sweating
    C   Craniotabes
    D   Coxa vara
    E   Premature closure of the anterior fontanelles

58. **Clinical features of idiopathic hypercalcaemia of infancy are:**
    A   Severe constipation
    B   Low serum cholesterol
    C   Short Q–T interval on electrocardiogram
    D   Irreversible mental retardation
    E   Hypertension

59. **Iron poisoning in children:**
A   Is less likely to occur with ferrous gluconate than with ferrous sulphate
B   May produce melaena stools
C   May produce jaundice
D   Commonly produces cardiac failure
E   Produces respiratory acidosis

60. **The following changes are typical of adrenaline as compared to noradrenaline:**
A   Lower chance of developing hyperglycaemia
B   More marked elevation of the blood pressure
C   More marked increase in peripheral resistance
D   Marked increase in cardiac output
E   More marked action on free fatty acid release

189

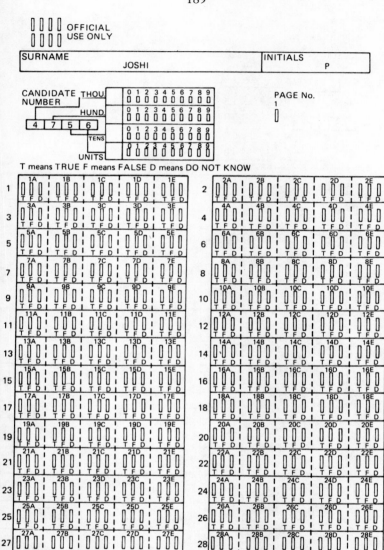

OFFICIAL USE ONLY

| SURNAME | JOSHI | INITIALS | P |

CANDIDATE NUMBER

THOU. 0 1 2 3 4 5 6 7 8 9

HUND. 0 1 2 3 4 5 6 7 8 9

4 7 5 6

TENS 0 1 2 3 4 5 6 7 8 9

UNITS 0 1 2 3 4 5 6 7 8 9

PAGE No. 1

T means TRUE F means FALSE D means DO NOT KNOW

190

SURNAME	INITIALS
JOSHI	P

CANDIDATE NUMBER

THOU. 0 1 2 3 4 5 6 7 8 9

HUND. 0 1 2 3 4 5 6 7 8 9

4 7 5 6

TENS 0 1 2 3 4 5 6 7 8 9

UNITS 0 1 2 3 4 5 6 7 8 9

PAGE No.
1

T means TRUE F means FALSE D means DO NOT KNOW

Answer grid with rows numbered 31 to 60, columns A–E, each with T F D options.

Answers to Examination 9
(For complete References see Chapter 3)

1. A True
    B False
    C True
    D True
    E False
    Other causes include:
    Nezelof syndrome
    Hodgkin's disease
    Lepromatous leprosy
    Ataxia telangiectasia
    Lymphosarcoma
    Chronic mucocutaneous
    candidiasis
    Secondary syphilis
    Severe burns
    Advanced malignancy
    Advanced rheumatoid
    arthritis
    Malnutrition
    Pyoderma gangraenosum,
    etc
    Ref. (2) pp. 319–320, 325

2. A False (prolonged)
    B True
    C False
    D True
    E False
    Ref. (11) p. 298

3. A False
    B False
    C False
    D False
    E True
    Ref. (10) pp. 398–401

4. A True
    B False (murmur is
       produced by
       pulmonary outflow
       tract obstruction; the
       ventricular septal
       defect is large and
       produces no
       murmurs)
    C False
    D False (most
       uncommon)
    E False
    Ref. (10) pp. 309–313

5. A False
    B True
    C True
    D False
    E True
    Ref. (10) pp. 489–491

6. A True
    B False (anterior
       descending branch)
    C False
    D True
    E False (10%)
    Ref. (10) pp. 467–469

7. A True
    B False
    C False
    D True
    E True
    Ref. (1) pp. 183–184

192

8. A   True
    B   True
    C   False
        (hypoprothrombin-
        aemia)
    D   True
    E   False
    Ref. (1) pp. 167–169

9. A   False (recessive)
    B   True
    C   True
    D   False
    E   True
    Ref. (1) pp. 156–157

10. A   False (late 60s)
    B   True
    C   True
    D   False (high)
    E   False (normal)
    Ref. (1) pp. 159–160

11. A   False
    B   False
    C   True
    D   False
    E   True
    Ref. (9) p. 155

12. A   False (about 5%)
    B   True
    C   True
    D   False
    E   True
    Ref. (9) p. 77

13. A   False
    B   True
    C   True
    D   True
    E   False
    Ref. (9) p. 250

14. A   False
    B   True
    C   True
    D   True
    E   False
    Ref. (9) p. 21

15. A   True
    B   True
    C   False
    D   False
    E   False
    Killed organisms also used
    in:
    Paratyphoid A and B,
    Cholera, Rabies, Anthrax,
    Influenza, Pertussis.
    Live attenuated organisms
    used in:
    Sabin vaccine
    (poliomyelitis),
    Smallpox,
    Yellow fever,
    Influenza.
    Toxoids used in:
    Diphtheria
    Tetanus
    Ref. (49) pp. 210–213

16. A   True
    B   True
    C   True
    D   True
    E   False (may occur
        rarely)
    Ref. (53) pp. 677–682

17. A   False (idiopathic)
    B   False
    C   True (wave and
        spike pattern at
        3 cycles/second)
    D   True
    E   False
    Ref. (53) p. 881

18. A True
    B True (during the early stages)
    C True
    D False
    E False
    Ref. (53) p. 909

19. A True
    B False
    C False (anterior osseus nerve affected)
    D True
    E True
    Ref. (53) pp. 452–453

20. A True
    B True (most reliable)
    C True (in one-third of patients)
    D False (bradycardia)
    E False
    Ref. (2) pp. 821–822

21. A False
    B True
    C False
    D False (20–30%)
    E True
    Ref. (2) pp. 807–871

22. A True
    B True
    C True
    D False (rare)
    E False (rare)
    Ref. (2) pp. 736–737

23. A False
    B True
    C True
    D True
    E False
    Ref. (2) pp. 1405–1406
         (4)

24. A True
    B True
    C False
    D False
    E True
    Ref. (2) p. 1420

25. A False (relieved)
    B True
    C True
    D False
    E False
    Ref. (2) pp. 1422–1423

26. A True
    B True
    C True
    D False
    E False
    Ref. (2) p. 694

27. A True
    B True
    C True
    D True
    E True
    Ref. (2) pp. 1647–1653

28. A True
    B False
    C True
    D False (difficulty in micturition)
    E True
    Ref. (6) pp. 121–128

29. A True
    B True
    C True
    D False
    E False
    Ref. (6) p. 639

30. A False
    B True
    C True
    D True
    E True
    Ref. (6) pp. 768–774

31. A True
    B False
    C True
    D False
    E False
    Ref. (6) pp. 327–328

32. A False
    B True
    C True
    D False
    E True
    Ref. (2) pp. 333, 335, 1337

33. A False (unusual;
       neurological
       involvement also
       unusual)
    B True
    C True
    D False
    E True
    Ref. (2) p. 159

34. A True
    B True
    C False
    D False
    E True
    Ref. (2) pp. 1701–1703

35. A True
    B False
    C True
    D False
    E True
    Ref. (2) p. 1766

36. A True
    B True
    C False
    D True
    E True
    Ref. (2) p. 475

37. A True
    B False
    C False
    D True
    E True
    Ref. (5) p. 193

38. A True
    B True
    C True
    D False
    E False
    Ref. (5) p. 196

39. A False
    B True
    C False
       (hyperthyroidism)
    D False (hypocalcaemia
       produced)
    E True
    Ref. (5) p. 189

40. A True
    B True (usually in
       chronic haemolysis)
    C True
    D True
    E False
       (hyperparathyroidism
    Ref. (5) pp. 189–190

41. A   True
    B   False
    C   True
    D   False
    E   True
    Ref. (25) p. 1007

42. A   False
    B   True
    C   True
    D   True
    E   False
    Ref. (23) p. 144

43. A   True
    B   False (more likely)
    C   False (equal to or greater than zero)
    D   True
    E   True
    Ref. (17)

44. A   False
    B   False
    C   True
    D   False
    E   True
    Ref. (24) p. 150

45. A   True (80%)
    B   True
    C   True
    D   False
    E   False
    Ref. (3) pp. 53–55

46. A   False
    B   True
    C   False
    D   True
    E   True
    Ref. (8) pp. 168–170, 943

47. A   True
    B   True
    C   False
    D   True
    E   False
    Ref. (8) pp. 188–190

48. A   True
    B   True
    C   False
    D   True
    E   False
    Ref. (8) p. 1200

49. A   True
    B   False
    C   False
    D   False
    E   True
    Ref. (8) pp. 1193–1195

50. A   False
    B   True
    C   True (delayed in coagulation defects)
    D   True
    E   False
    Ref. (8) p. 1206

51. A   False
    B   False (unaffected)
    C   True
    D   True
    E   False
    Ref. (8) pp. 1208–1210

52. A   True
    B   True
    C   True
    D   False
    E   False
    Ref. (8) pp. 1413–1416

53. A   True
    B   False (15–25 years)
    C   True
    D   False
    E   True
    Ref. (*19*) pp. 405–407

54. A   False
    B   True
    C   True
    D   False (upper extremities)
    E   True
    Ref. (*19*) pp. 369–371

55. A   True
    B   False
    C   True
    D   True
    E   False
    Ref. (*19*) pp. 309–313

56. A   True
    B   False
    C   False
    D   True
    E   True
    Ref. (*15*) pp. 283–306

57. A   False (hypotonia)
    B   True
    C   True
    D   True
    E   False
    Ref. (*15*) p. 579

58. A   True
    B   False (increased)
    C   True
    D   True
    E   True
    Ref. (*15*) p. 593

59. A   True
    B   True
    C   True
    D   False
    E   False
    Ref. (*15*) pp. 629–630

60. A   False
    B   True
    C   False
    D   True
    E   False
    Ref. (*21*) p. 279

Examination 10
(Time allotted: 2½ hours)

1. **In bicuspid aortic valves:**
   A   Coarctation of the aorta may be associated
   B   Calcification of the valves is uncommon
   C   Infective endocarditis is very uncommon
   D   Incompetence is more constantly present than stenosis
   E   There is a high association with Turner's syndrome

2. **High output cardiac failure is recognized in:**
   A   Primary hyperparathyroidism
   B   Ruptured sinus of Valsalva
   C   Ventricular septal defect
   D   Liver failure
   E   Cor pulmonale

3. **In aortic arteritis (Takayasu's disease):**
   A   The carotid sinuses are abnormally sensitive
   B   Visual symptoms are prominent
   C   Heart failure is rare
   D   Claudication of the jaws may occur
   E   Bowel ischaemia is uncommon

4. **A loud 1st heart sound is found in:**
   A Complete heart block
   B Severe mitral incompetence
   C Mitral stenosis
   D Acute myocarditis
   E Large pulmonary embolus

5. **Characteristic physical signs of a large pneumo-thorax include:**
   A Dullness to percussion of the affected side
   B Reduced breath sounds on the affected side
   C End-inspiratory crepitations
   D Contralateral shift of the mediastinum
   E Impaired chest movements on the affected side

6. **Treatment of status asthmaticus includes:**
   A 40% oxygen if the Pa_{CO_2} is increased
   B Sedation with pethidine if the patient is very restless
   C Intravenous hydrocortisone
   D Salbutamol spray inhalations
   E Restriction of fluids to avoid cardiac failure

7. **In the differentiation between chronic bronchitis and pure emphysema, the following may be of value:**
   A Wheezing and rhonchi
   B Pa_{CO_2}
   C Diffusing capacity
   D Pa_{O_2}
   E Blood eosinophilia

8. **The following factors predispose to the development of thromboembolism:**
   A Carcinoma of the pancreas
   B Blood group O
   C Oral contraceptives
   D Obesity
   E Myocardial infarction

9. **Porphyria cutanea tarda symptomatica is characterized by:**
   A   An inherited predisposition
   B   Marked photosensitivity
   C   Severe reactions following barbiturates
   D   Exacerbation of skin symptoms after chloroquine administration
   E   Markedly increased urinary excretion of uroporphyrins only

10. **Drug-induced jaundice is produced by:**
   A   Phenelzine
   B   Phenylbutazone
   C   Penicillin sensitivity reactions
   D   Chlordiazepoxide
   E   Novobiocin

11. **Conditions predisposing to carcinoma of the colon are:**
   A   Ulcerative colitis
   B   Chronic giardiasis
   C   Familial multiple polyposis
   D   Regional ileitis (Crohn's disease)
   E   Hirschsprung's disease

12. **Acute diverticulitis may present with:**
   A   Alternating constipation and diarrhoea
   B   Severe rectal haemorrhage
   C   Vitamin B_{12} deficiency anaemia
   D   Subacute obstruction
   E   Melaena stools

13. **In hydatid disease:**
   A   Mainly the right lobe of the liver is involved
   B   The brain may be affected
   C   Multiple cysts are typically produced in the liver
   D   Treatment is percutaneous needle aspiration of the liver
   E   Cysts in the long bone usually necessitate amputation

14. **The medial cord of the brachial plexus gives off the following branches:**
    A Nerve to latissimus dorsi
    B Ulnar nerve
    C A root to the median nerve
    D Radial nerve
    E Musculocutaneous nerve

15. **The Arnold–Chiari malformation:**
    A May produce hydrocephalus
    B Is often associated with syringomyelia
    C May be associated with lumbosacral spina bifida
    D Is associated with congenital heart lesions
    E May produce bladder dysfunction

16. **Dysphasia is caused by:**
    A Left temporal lobe abscess
    B Alzheimer's disease
    C Parkinson's syndrome
    D Motor neurone disease
    E Intracranial tumour

17. **A decreased glucose and an increased protein in the cerebrospinal fluid is produced by:**
    A Tuberculosis
    B Cryptococcal meningitis
    C Carcinomatous meningitis
    D Sarcoid meningitis
    E Coxsackie meningitis

18. **The following features suggest a subarachnoid haemorrhage as opposed to a traumatic lumbar puncture:**
    A Increased cerebrospinal fluid pressure
    B Bloody mixture in the initial collecting tubes only
    C Failure of the collected fluid to clot
    D Crenated red cells under the microscope
    E Raised lactic dehydrogenase levels in the cerebrospinal fluid

19. **The following urinary values are normal:**
   A   Proteins of 0.3 g/24 hours
   B   Red cells of 1 000 000/24 hours
   C   Casts of 300 000/24 hours
   D   Urobilinogen of 12 mg/24 hours
   E   pH of 4.6–8.0

20. **Analgesic nephropathy:**
   A   Produces a typical picture on intravenous pyelography
   B   Progresses despite stopping the ingestion of the causative agent
   C   May present as a chronic pyelonephritis-like disease
   D   May produce anuria
   E   May be produced by chronic codeine ingestion

21. **Damage to the S_2–S_4 segments of the cord:**
   A   May be caused by poliomyelitis
   B   May be caused by tabes dorsalis
   C   Produces a large capacity bladder
   D   Produces involuntary detrusor contractions
   E   Produces marked bladder trabeculations

22. **A hypernephroma may present with:**
   A   Pyrexia of unexplained aetiology
   B   High output failure
   C   Hypocalcaemia
   D   Hypotension
   E   Nephrotic syndrome

23. **A monoclonal gammopathy is found with:**
   A   Systemic lupus erythematosus
   B   Sarcoidosis
   C   Myeloma
   D   Macroglobulinaemia
   E   Benign paraproteinaemia

24. **Urinary calcium loss is increased in:**
    A   Osteoporosis
    B   Osteomalacia
    C   Primary hyperparathyroidism
    D   Secondary hyperparathyroidism
    E   Sarcoidosis

25. **Hypocomplementaemia is seen in:**
    A   Acute rheumatic fever
    B   Paroxysmal nocturnal haemoglobinuria
    C   Nephritis complicating an infected ventriculoatrial shunt
    D   Membranoproliferative glomerulonephritis
    E   Acute poststreptococcal nephritis

26. **Electrocardiographic changes of hyperkalaemia include:**
    A   Tall 'u' waves
    B   Absent 'p' waves
    C   Wide QRS complexes
    D   Ventricular tachycardia
    E   Depressed ST segments

27. **The disadvantages of premature birth are:**
    A   Higher incidence of intracranial haemorrhage
    B   Inadequate sweating leading to hyperthermia
    C   Respiratory centre immaturity
    D   Inadequate vitamin B_{12} levels producing anaemia
    E   Increased susceptibility to infections

28. **The idiopathic respiratory distress syndrome is predisposed to by:**
    A   Antepartum haemorrhage
    B   Maternal alveolar proteinosis
    C   Caesarian section
    D   Maternal diabetes mellitus
    E   Maternal steroid therapy

29. **Umbilical sepsis:**
   A   Is most often due to *Staphylococcus aureus*
   B   Is usually severe
   C   May present with multiple abscesses in the liver
   D   Not uncommonly produces direct spread to the peritoneal cavity
   E   Requires systemic antibiotic therapy in most patients

30. **In acute bronchiolitis of infancy:**
   A   The temperature is commonly about 104°F (40°C)
   B   Bilateral obstructive emphysema is produced
   C   The chest x-ray is diagnostic
   D   The mortality rate is about 50%
   E   The spleen is occasionally palpable

31. **The following features are compatible with a myelophthisic anaemia:**
   A   Howell–Jolly bodies on the peripheral smear
   B   Increased nucleated red cells on the peripheral smear
   C   White cell count of 26 000/mm^3
   D   Thrombocytosis
   E   Demonstration of the primary disease on the bone marrow

32. **Thymic tumours are associated with:**
   A   Myasthenia gravis
   B   Congenital hypogammaglobulinaemia
   C   Cushing's syndrome
   D   Marked pancytopenia
   E   Folate deficiency anaemia

33. **In thalassaemia major:**
   A   Fetal haemoglobin may be up to 90% of the total
   B   A value of 35% target cells on the smear is diagnostic
   C   Splenomegaly is present
   D   Haemoglobin A is decreased
   E   Haemoglobin A$_2$ is increased

34. **Homocystinuria:**
    A   Is due to an inborn error of methionine metabolism
    B   Is indistinguishable from Marfan's syndrome
    C   Typically produces hepatosplenomegaly
    D   Produces an increased incidence of venous thrombosis
    E   Produces a positive nitroprusside screening test

35. **The following features suggest hypomania as opposed to anxiety:**
    A   Pressure of talk
    B   Apprehensive and fearful
    C   Overconfident and grandiose
    D   Tense posture
    E   Alert and jumpy

36. **Delirium tremens is characterized by:**
    A   Marked somnolence
    B   A gradual onset
    C   Visual hallucinations
    D   Bradycardia
    E   Illusions

37. **Loss of appetite or refusal of food in a 3-year-old child may be a result of:**
    A   Early schizophrenia
    B   Negativistic behaviour
    C   Daydreaming
    D   Anorexia nervosa
    E   Parental oversolicitude

38. **Anorexia nervosa is characterized by:**
    A   A history of induced vomiting
    B   Lethargy and tiredness
    C   Hirsutism
    D   Menorrhagia
    E   Periods of having a ravenous appetite and overeating

39. **Erythema multiforme:**
  A Is commonly caused by a viral infection
  B May be produced by *Mycoplasma pneumoniae*
  C Usually requires systemic steroid therapy
  D May be associated with sarcoidosis
  E May sometimes be a result of steroid usage

40. **Syphilis is known to produce the following skin lesions:**
  A Copper coloured bullous lesions
  B Unilateral hyperkeratosis of the sole
  C Condylomata accuminata
  D Mucocutaneous lesions
  E Discrete punched out circinate ulcer

41. **Anticoagulants are known to interact with:**
  A Griseofulvin
  B Morphine
  C Phenobarbital
  D Paracetamol
  E Clofibrate (Atromid S)

42. **Chlorpromazine:**
  A Blocks the response to stimulation of the reticular activating system
  B Produces mydriasis
  C Produces a rise in the body temperature
  D Produces postural hypotension
  E Produces non-puerperal lactation

43. **ʟ-Dopa produces the following adverse reactions:**
  A Choreo-athetosis
  B Hypertension
  C Jaundice
  D Hallucinatory toxic psychosis
  E Diarrhoea

44. **Indications for steroid therapy include:**
   A   Atopic dermatitis
   B   Sarcoidosis
   C   Cushing's syndrome
   D   Pemphigoid
   E   Hereditary spherocytosis

45. **Diazoxide (Hyperstat):**
   A   Is chemically related to the thiazide diuretics
   B   Is of value in the treatment of insulin–producing tumours
   C   Can only be given intravenously
   D   Produces alopecia
   E   Is of value in the long–term management of hypertension

46. **Coarse crepitations are characteristically found in:**
   A   The early stages of pneumonia
   B   Fibrosing alveolitis
   C   Bronchiectasis
   D   Left ventricular failure
   E   Bronchitis

47. **Papilloedema is well recognized with:**
   A   Friedreich's ataxia
   B   Subarachnoid haemorrhage
   C   Acute meningitis
   D   Cerebellar tumours
   E   Tumours of the 4th ventricle

48. **Noonan's syndrome typically produces:**
   A   Tall stature
   B   Webbing of the neck
   C   Normal chromosomal pattern
   D   Cardiovascular abnormalities
   E   Gynaecomastia

49. **The clinical presentation of cretinism includes:**
   A   Obesity in the child
   B   Goitre in almost all patients
   C   Spastic diplegia
   D   Deafness
   E   Mental deficiency

50. **Deficiency of antidiuretic hormone may be due to:**
   A   Suprasellar tumours
   B   Healed tuberculous meningitis
   C   Marfan's syndrome
   D   Chronic renal failure
   E   Sarcoidosis

51. **Uric acid reabsorption is blocked by:**
   A   Low dose salicylates
   B   Hyperlacticacidaemia
   C   Phenylbutazone
   D   Dicoumarols
   E   Probenecid

52. **Radiological paraspinal calcification is caused by:**
   A   Fluorosis
   B   Psoriasis
   C   Hypoparathyroidism
   D   Familial hypophosphataemia
   E   Thyrotoxicosis

53. **A painful heel is caused by:**
   A   Ankylosing spondylitis
   B   Kohler's disease
   C   Rheumatoid arthritis
   D   Prolonged diazepam therapy
   E   Gonococcal infection

54. **Inflammatory arteritis is typically found with:**
   A   Polyarteritis nodosa
   B   Aortic arch syndrome
   C   Rheumatic fever
   D   Henoch–Schönlein purpura
   E   Endarteritis obliterans

55. **X-linked inheritance is described in:**
   A   Glucose-6-phosphate dehydrogenase deficiency
   B   Hurler's syndrome
   C   Pseudohypertrophic muscular dystrophy of
       Duchenne
   D   Lesch–Nyhan syndrome
   E   Vitamin D-resistant rickets

56. **Retrobulbar neuritis:**
   A   Typically produces an enlargement of the blind spot
   B   Is caused by disseminated sclerosis
   C   May be caused by the pentavalent tryparsamides
   D   May be caused by congenital toxoplasmosis
   E   Is rarely caused by vitamin B_{12} deficiency

57. **In rubella:**
   A   A morbilliform rash is produced
   B   Suboccipital lymphadenopathy is consistently
       found
   C   Lymphopenia occurs commonly
   D   Arthritis occurs
   E   Repeated attacks of rubella are not uncommon

58. **In smallpox:**
   A   The temperature rises further within 24 hours after
       the development of the rash
   B   The extent of the rash is a function of the severity
       of the disease
   C   The mortality rate may be up to 40%
   D   Antibiotics in the early stages are of great benefit
   E   Vaccinated contacts may develop a febrile illness
       without the rash

59. **The following statements are true:**
  A   The mean and standard deviation of a random sample will generally be different from the mean and standard deviation of the population
  B   If a given sample mean lies within the 66% range, it is 'consistent' with the population mean
  C   The sampling distribution of the mean will be normal if the parent population is itself normally distributed
  D   All the normal distribution curves are of different general shape and characteristics
  E   The size of the sample determines the dispersion of the sample means around the population mean

60. **Herpes simplex infection produces:**
  A   A high association with carcinoma of the uterus
  B   Kaposi's varicelliform eruption
  C   Keratoconjunctivitis
  D   Subacute sclerosing panencephalitis
  E   Acute gingivostomatitis

210

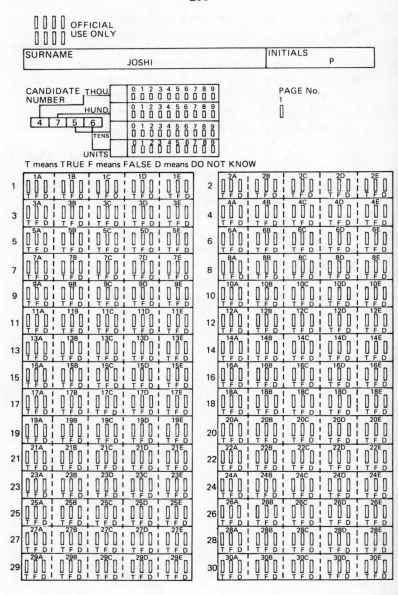

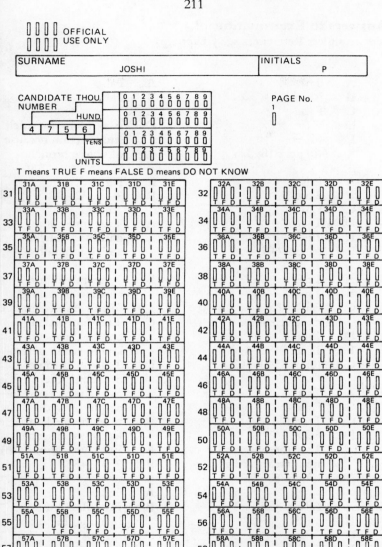

OFFICIAL USE ONLY

SURNAME: JOSHI

INITIALS: P

CANDIDATE NUMBER

THOU. 0 1 2 3 4 5 6 7 8 9
HUND. 0 1 2 3 4 5 6 7 8 9
4 7 5 6
TENS 0 1 2 3 4 5 6 7 8 9
UNITS 0 1 2 3 4 5 6 7 8 9

PAGE No. 1

T means TRUE F means FALSE D means DO NOT KNOW

Answers to Examination 10
(For complete References see Chapter 3)

1. A   True
   B   False
   C   False
   D   False
   E   False
   Ref. (*10*) pp. 318, 326

2. A   False
   B   True
   C   False
   D   True
   E   True
   Ref. (*10*) pp. 607–608

3. A   True
   B   True
   C   False (secondary to hypertension)
   D   True
   E   True
   Ref. (*10*) pp. 560–563

4. A   True
   B   False
   C   True
   D   False
   E   True (because of the sinus tachycardia)
   Ref. (*10*) pp. 57–59

5. A   False
   B   True
   C   False
   D   True
   E   True
   Ref. (*9*) p. 47

6. A   False
   B   False
   C   True
   D   False (does not reach site of action because of severe broncho- spasm)
   E   False
   Ref. (*9*) p. 132

7. A   True (present in chronic bronchitis; absent in emphy- sema)
   B   True (raised in chronic bronchitis; low in emphysema)
   C   True (normal in chronic bronchitis; low in emphysema)
   D   True (in chronic bronchitis the Pao_2 drops early; in emphysema the Pao_2 is maintained until late in the disease
   E   False (absent in both)
   Ref. (*9*) p. 146

8. A   True
   B   False (less common than in other blood groups)
   C   True (risk increased 6 times)
   D   True
   E   True (5% of patients)
   Ref. (*9*) pp. 162–164

9. A   True
    B   True
    C   False
    D   True
    E   True
    (aminolaevulinic
    acid and porpho-
    bilinogen not
    found)
    Ref. (*42*) pp. 327–328

10. A   True
    B   True
    C   True
    D   True
    E   True
    Ref. (*42*) p. 278

11. A   True
    B   False
    C   True
    D   False
    E   False
    Ref. (*12*) p. 517

12. A   True
    B   True
    C   False
    D   True
    E   False
    Ref. (*52*) pp. 326–327

13. A   True (75%)
    B   True
    C   False
    D   False
    E   True
    Ref. (*52*) pp. 789–790

14. A   False (from posterior
    cord)
    B   True
    C   True
    D   False (from posterior
    cord)
    E   False (from lateral
    cord)
    Ref. (*14*) pp. 225–228

15. A   True
    B   True
    C   True
    D   False
    E   False
    Ref. (*26*) pp. 234, 238, 333

16. A   True
    B   True
    C   False
    D   False
    E   True
    Ref. (*26*) p. 122

17. A   True
    B   True
    C   True
    D   True
    E   False
    Ref. (*4*) p. 180

18. A   True
    B   False
    C   True
    D   True (due to the
    higher chloride
    concentration in the
    cerebrospinal fluid)
    E   False
    Ref. (*4*) p. 176

19. A   False
     (0.1 g/24 hours)
  B   True
  C   False (up to
     100 000/24 hours)
  D   False
     (0–4 mg/24 hours)
  E   True
Ref. (4) p. 13

20. A   True
  B   False
  C   True
  D   True
  E   False
Ref. (5) pp. 35–36

21. A   True
  B   True
  C   True
  D   False
  E   False
Ref. (5) p. 168

22. A   True
  B   True (multiple
     arteriovenous
     fistulae may develop
     within the tumour)
  C   False
     (hypercalcaemia;
     also polycythaemia
     or Cushing's
     syndrome)
  D   False (hypertension)
  E   True
Ref. (5) pp. 164–165

23. A   False
  B   False
  C   True
  D   True
  E   True
Ref. (5) p. 190

24. A   False (normal)
  B   False (decreased)
  C   True
  D   False (decreased)
  E   True
Ref. (5) p. 191

25. A   False
  B   False
  C   True
  D   True
  E   True
Ref. (5) p. 194

26. A   False (seen in
     hypokalaemia)
  B   True
  C   True
  D   True
  E   False
Ref. (11) p. 95

27. A   True
  B   False
  C   True
  D   False
  E   True
Ref. (15) pp. 14–15

28. A   True
  B   False
  C   True
  D   True
  E   False
Ref. (15) p. 21

29. A   True
  B   False
  C   True
  D   False (excessively
     rare)
  E   False
Ref. (15) p. 90

30. A   False
     B   True
     C   False
     D   False (5%)
     E   True
     Ref. (15) p. 245
         (8) p. 862

31. A   False
     B   True
     C   True
     D   False
     E   True
     Ref. (4) p. 210

32. A   True
     B   True
     C   True
     D   False
     E   False
     Ref. (4) p. 213

33. A   True
     B   False
     C   True
     D   True
     E   False
     Ref. (4) pp. 222–223

34. A   True
     B   False
     C   False
     D   True
     E   True
     Ref. (4) p. 264

35. A   True
     B   False
     C   True
     D   False
     E   False
     Ref. (35) p. 182

36. A   False (insomnia)
     B   False (sudden onset)
     C   True
     D   False
     E   True
     Ref. (35) p. 234

37. A   False
     B   True
     C   True
     D   False
     E   True
     Ref. (35) pp. 269–270

38. A   True
     B   False (paradoxically active)
     C   False
     D   False (amenorrhoea)
     E   True
     Ref. (35) pp. 127–128

39. A   True (Herpes simplex infection in one-third of cases)
     B   True
     C   False
     D   False
     E   False
     Ref. (3) pp. 126, 199
         (2) pp. 190, 245, 386, 1651

40. A   True (congenital syphilis)
     B   True (tertiary syphilis—a rare manifestation)
     C   False
     D   True
     E   True (gumma)
     Ref. (3) p. 75

41. A True
     B False
     C True
     D False
     E True
     Ref. (*7*) p. 158

42. A False
     B True
     C False
     D True
     E True
     Ref. (*7*) p. 225

43. A True
     B False (hypotension)
     C False
     D True
     E False
     Ref. (*7*) pp. 287–288

44. A True
     B True
     C False
     D False
     E False
     Ref. (*7*) p. 324
           (*39*)

45. A True
     B True
     C False (oral tablets
        also)
     D False (hirsutism)
     E False
     Ref. (*7*) p. 345

46. A False
     B True
     C True
     D False
     E True
     Ref. (*13*) pp. 184–185

47. A False
     B True
     C False (subacute or
        chronic more
        commonly)
     D True
     E True
     Ref. (*13*) pp. 397–399

48. A False (short stature)
     B True
     C True
     D True
     E False
     Ref. (*47*) pp. 103–104

49. A False
     B False
     C True
     D True
     E True
     Ref. (*16*) p. 70

50. A True
     B True
     C False
     D False
     E True
     Ref. (*16*) p. 24

51. A False (blocks
        secretions)
     B False (blocks
        secretions)
     C True
     D True
     E True
     Ref. (*1*) p. 133

52.   A   True
     B   True
     C   True
     D   True
     E   False
     Also true for:
     Reiter's disease
     Paraplegia
     Still's disease
     Ulcerative colitis
     Crohn's disease
     Whipple's disease
     Baastrup's disease (senile
     ankylosing hyperostosis)
     Ankylosing spondylitis
     Ref. (1) p. 110

53.   A   True
     B   False (osteochond-
          ritis of the 2nd
          metatarsal head)
     C   True
     D   False
     E   True
     Ref. (1) p. 162

54.   A   True
     B   False
          (non-inflammatory
          arteritis)
     C   True
     D   True
     E   False
          (non-inflammatory
          arteritis seen with
          rheumatoid arthritis
          and progressive
          systemic sclerosis)
     Ref. (1) p. 93

55.   A   True
     B   False (autosomal
          recessive)
     C   True
     D   True
     E   True (x-linked
          dominant)
     Ref. (25) pp. 1007–1008

56.   A   False
     B   True
     C   True
     D   False
     E   True
     Ref. (24) p. 265

57.   A   True
     B   True
     C   False
     D   True
     E   False
     Ref. (2) pp. 795–797

58.   A   False
     B   True
     C   True
     D   False
     E   True
     Ref. (8) pp. 126–131

59.   A   True
     B   False (95%)
     C   True
     D   False
     E   True
     Ref. (17)

60.   A   False (carcinoma of
          the cervix)
     B   True
     C   True
     D   False
     E   True
     Ref. (8) pp. 158–160

Chapter 3
Bibliographical References to the Answers

(1) Dick, W. C. (1977). *An Introduction to Clinical Rheumatology*. New York: Churchill Livingstone
(2) *Harrison's Principles of Internal Medicine* (1980). 9th edn. New York: McGraw-Hill
(3) Sneddon, I. B. and Church, R. E. (1982). *Practical Dermatology*. 4th edn. London: Arnold
(4) Wallach, J. (1970). *Interpretation of Diagnostic Tests*. Boston: Little, Brown & Co.
(5) Gabriel, R. (1975). *Postgraduate Nephrology*. London: Butterworths
(6) Goodman, L. S. and Gilman, A. (1980). *The Pharmacological Basis of Therapeutics*. 6th edn. New York: Macmillan
(7) Meyers, F. H., Jawetz, E. and Goldfien, A. (1970). *Review of Medical Pharmacology*. 2nd edn. California: Lange
(8) Bodley Scott, R. (1978). *Price's Textbook of the Practice of Medicine*. 12th edn. London: Oxford University Press
(9) Schonnell, M. (1978). *Respiratory Medicine*. New York: Churchill Livingstone
(10) Schrire, V. (1971). *Clinical Cardiology*. 3rd edn. London: Staples Press
(11) Schamroth, L. (1982). *An Introduction to Electrocardiography*. 6th edn. London: Blackwell
(12) Jawetz, E., Melnick, J. L. and Adelberg, E. A. (1970). *Review of Medical Microbiology*. 9th edn. California: Lange
(13) Swash, M. and Mason, S. (1984). *Hutchison's Clinical Methods*. 18th edn. London: Baillière Tindall
(14) Ellis, H. (1983). *Clinical Anatomy*. 7th edn. London: Blackwell
(15) Hutchison, J. H. (1980). *Practical Paediatric Problems*. 5th edn. London: Lloyd-Luke

(16) Thomson, J. A. (1981). *An Introduction to Clinical Endocrinology.* 2nd edn. New York: Churchill Livingstone

(17) Bourke, G. J. and McGilvray, J. (1975). *Interpretation and Uses of Medical Statistics.* 2nd edn. London: Blackwell

(18) Davies, L. J. T. (1972). *Postgraduate Medicine.* 2nd edn. London: Lloyd-Luke

(19) Kolb, L. C. (1977). *Noyes' Modern Clinical Psychiatry.* 9th edn. New York: Saunders

(20) Rubinstein, D. and Mayne, D. (1983). *Lecture Notes on Clinical Medicine.* 2nd edn. London: Blackwell

(21) Ganong, M. F. (1979). *Review of Medical Physiology.* 9th edn. California: Lange

(22) Ogilvie, G. M. (1980). *Chamberlain's Symptoms and Signs in Clinical Medicine.* 10th edn. Bristol: Wright

(23) Vaughan, D. and Asbury, T. (1983). *General Ophthalmology.* 10th edn. California: Lange

(24) Pappworth, M. M. (1984). *A Primer of Medicine.* 5th edn. London: Butterworths

(25) Kempe, C. H., Silver, H. K. and O'Brien, D. (1984). *Current Pediatric Diagnosis and Treatment.* 8th edn. California: Lange

(26) Bannister, R. (1981). *Brain's Clinical Neurology.* 5th edn. London: Oxford University Press

(27) Sherlock, S. (1981). *Diseases of the Liver and Biliary System.* 6th edn. London: Blackwell

(28) *British Journal of Hospital Medicine*

(a)	(December, 1978)	Volume 20/6
(b)	(March, 1978)	Volume 19/3
(c)	(November, 1977)	Volume 18/5
(d)	(December, 1977)	Volume 18/6
(e)	(September, 1978)	Volume 20/3
(f)	(October, 1978)	Volume 20/4
(g)	(June, 1978)	Volume 19/6
(h)	(April, 1978)	Volume 19/4
(i)	(March, 1979)	Volume 21/3
(j)	(February, 1978)	Volume 19/2
(k)	(July, 1979)	Volume 22/1

(29) Robinson, R. and Stott, R. (1977). *Medical Emergencies, Diagnosis and Management.* 2nd edn. London: Heinemann

(30) The Medical Clinics of North America (November 1977). *Pulmonary Disease.* Vol. 61, Number 6. New York: Saunders

(31) Foxen, E. H. M. (1972). *Lecture Notes on the Diseases of the Ear, Nose and Throat.* 3rd edn. London: Blackwell

(32) Guyton, A. C. (1981). *Textbook of Medical Physiology.* 6th edn. Philadelphia: Saunders

(33) Turk, J. L. (1972). *Immunology in Clinical Medicine.* 2nd edn. London: Heinemann

(*34*) de Wardener, M. E. (1973). *The Kidney*. 4th edn. London: Churchill

(*35*) Linford Rees, W. L. (1980). *A Short Textbook of Psychiatry*. 2nd edn. London: English University Press

(*36*) Batchelor, I. R. C. (1978). *Henderson and Gillespie's Textbook of Psychiatry*. 10th edn. London: Oxford University Press

(*37*) Thomas, B. A., *Immunology*. The Upjohn Company Monograph. Michigan, USA

(*38*) Wood, P. (1968). *Diseases of the Heart and Circulation*. 3rd edn. London: Eyre and Spottiswoode

(*39*) Daggett, P.R. and Geddes, D.M. (1976). *Practical Medicine: A Guide to Out-patient Management*. London: Lloyd–Luke

(*40*) Crofton, J. and Douglas, A. (1975). *Respiratory Diseases*. 2nd edn. Oxford: Blackwell

(*41*) Read, A. E. *et al.* (1967). Neuropsychiatric syndromes associated with chronic liver disease. *Quarterly Journal of Medicine*, Vol. 36

(*42*) Zilva, J. F. and Pannall, P. R. (1973). *Clinical Chemistry in Diagnosis and Treatment*. London: Lloyd–Luke

(*43*) Walton, J. N. (1977). *Brain's Diseases of the Nervous System*. 8th edn. Oxford: University Press

(*44*) Sutton, D. (1975). *A Textbook of Radiology*. 2nd edn. Edinburgh: Churchill Livingstone

(*45*) *Modern Medicine* (July 1979). South Africa, Vol. 4, No. 7:
   (*a*) Grand, H. G. and Lobes, Jr., L. A., Diabetes and the eye: recognizing problems early
   (*b*) Esterly, N. B. and Koransky, J. S., How to curb 14 familiar skin disorders in children

(*46*) Oriel, J. D. and Schachter, J. (1977). *Non-gonococcal Urethritis; The Most Common Venereal Disease*. Lederle Laboratories Issue

(*47*) Williams, R. H. (1981). *Textbook of Endocrinology*. 6th edn. Philadelphia: Saunders

(*48*) Boss, Seegmiller (28.6.1979). Hyperuricaemia and gout: classification, complications and management. *New England Journal of Medicine*. Vol. 300, No. 26

(*49*) Roitt, I. (1977). *Essential Immunology*. 3rd edn. London: Blackwell

(*50*) Azzopardi. J. G. (1968). *Carcinoma-Endocrine Syndrome*. 4th Symposium on Advanced Medicine. London: Pitman

(*51*) *British Medical Association Memorandum on Accidental Hypothermia in the Elderly* (1964). London

(*52*) Macleod, J. (1984). *Davidson's Principles and Practice of Medicine*, 14th edn. London: Churchill Livingstone

(*53*) Adams, R. D. and Victor, M. (1977). *Principles of Neurology*. New York: McGraw-Hill

(*54*) Fleckenstein, A. and Roskamm, H. (1980). *Calcium-Antagonismus*. International Symposium. Berlin: Springer Verlag

(*55*) Houstan, J. C., Joiner, C. L. and Trounce, J. R. (1979). *A Short Textbook of Medicine*. 6th edn. London: Unibooks

(*56*) Wilson, A. and Schild, H. O. (1968). *Applied Pharmacology*. 10th edn. London: Churchill

(*57*) *Monthly Index of Medical Specialities (MIMS) Desk Reference*. (1978–1979). Vol. 14, Pretoria, South Africa: Mims (PTY) Ltd.

(*58*) Vakil, R. J. and Golwalla, A. F., *Physical Diagnosis*. 1st edn. Bombay: Media Promoters and Publishers

(*59*) Wyngaarden, J. B. and Smith, L. H. (1982). *Cecil—Textbook of Medicine*. 16th edn. Philadelphia: Saunders

Chapter 4
Subject-Orientated Index
(A chapter dealing with cross-references to individual subjects so that all the multiple choice questions dealing with a particular subject can be collated and attempted if so desired.)

Metabolic diseases
Examination
1 Q. 1, 10, 16
2   8, 37, 48
3   2, 28, 42
4   30, 35
5   15, 21, 26, 27, 31, 51
6   47, 51, 53, 54
7   8, 15, 19, 54, 55
8   13, 16
9   11, 37, 39, 40, 57, 58
10   9, 24, 26, 34, 51

Respiratory diseases
Examination
1 Q. 2, 15, 29, 34, 55
2   16, 43, 44, 46, 55
3   17, 22, 31, 41, 43, 54
4   1, 14, 16, 19, 37, 45
5   2, 8, 17, 45, 50
6   1, 5, 6, 7, 8
7   1, 2, 3, 4, 13, 48, 52
8   5, 6, 7, 8, 14, 30
9   12, 13, 14, 31
10   5, 6, 7, 8, 30, 46

Collagen disorders
Examination
1 Q. 3, 8, 39, 42
2   17, 44
3   5, 9, 20, 23, 28, 48
5   12, 13
8   12, 33
9   7, 33
10   52, 53, 54

Dermatology
Examination
1 Q. 4, 7
2   2, 11, 14, 15, 46, 50
3   1, 3, 8, 20, 25
4   3, 5, 59
5   13, 16
6   23, 58, 59
7   53
8   53
9   27, 44, 45
10   39, 40, 57, 58

Haematology
Examination
1 Q. 5, 23, 26
2   18, 45, 56
3   7, 13, 16, 25
4   26, 40, 46, 49
5   7, 46, 47, 59
6   20, 21, 22, 48, 49, 55
7   7, 22, 31, 32, 33, 56
8   18, 19, 55, 56, 57
9   49, 50, 51
10   31, 33

Nephrology
Examination
1 Q. 6, 8, 57
2   23, 26, 32, 33, 40
3   32, 40, 52
4   27, 28, 29
5   1, 3, 43, 44, 55
6   43, 44, 45
7   25, 26, 27, 29
8   50, 51, 52
9   32, 36, 37, 38
10   19, 20, 22, 24

Infections and infectious disorders
Examination
1 Q. 2, 7, 14, 30, 46
2   20, 38, 47, 50
3   14, 49, 50, 51, 54, 55
4   23, 57, 58, 59
5   16, 20, 47, 52, 53, 54
6   24, 57, 58
7   46, 47, 48, 49, 50, 57
8   2, 5, 23, 29, 45, 46, 47, 49, 54
9   12, 20, 21, 22, 45, 47
10   13, 29, 30, 40, 57, 58, 60

Pharmacology
Examination
1 Q. 4, 9, 17, 41, 45, 52
2   10, 12, 23, 27, 30, 51
3   12, 13, 19, 27, 44, 45, 53
4   11, 22, 43, 53
5   8, 25, 38, 40, 44, 57, 58
6   33, 34, 35, 36, 37
7   5, 6, 7, 8, 9, 37, 45
8   15, 20, 21, 22, 23, 24, 25, 48
9   5, 8, 26, 28, 29, 30, 31, 33, 34
10   10, 41, 42, 43, 44, 45, 51

Venereal diseases
Examination
1 Q. 11
2   47
3   53
4   23, 47
5   20
6   4, 24
7   57
8   49
9   46
10   40

Gastroenterology
Examination
1 Q. 12, 36, 40, 49, 56
2   9, 19, 24, 28, 29, 30, 35, 49, 58
3   4, 10, 18, 29, 56
4   3, 4, 11, 12, 20, 21, 24, 36, 55
5   10, 11, 32, 37, 48, 49
6   9, 10, 11, 12, 15, 27
7   9, 16, 17, 18, 19, 31, 43
8   15, 16, 32, 33, 34, 35, 36, 37, 46, 59
9   23, 24, 25, 26, 38, 44
10   10, 11, 12, 13, 29, 38

Endocrinology
Examination
1   Q. 13, 24, 25, 32, 44, 58
2   10, 13, 25, 52
3   28, 35, 39
4   10, 31, 44, 56
5   9, 24, 25, 26
6   36, 40, 41, 42
7   14, 15, 19
8   9, 10, 11
9   34, 35
10   49

Neurology
Examination
1   Q. 16, 18, 19, 22, 47, 48,
       51, 53
2   2, 3, 4, 21, 50, 53, 59
3   6, 22, 33, 40, 45, 58
4   32, 33, 34, 41, 42, 48,
       57
5   7, 11, 14, 15, 18, 19,
       28, 34, 35
6   13, 16, 17, 18, 19, 29,
       40, 46, 56
7   14, 21, 23, 24, 34, 35,
       36, 37, 39, 41, 51, 59
8   9, 20, 26, 27, 28, 29,
       31, 39, 40
9   16, 17, 18, 19, 42, 54,
       55
10   14, 15, 16, 17, 18, 21,
       36, 47, 50, 56

Cardiology
Examination
1   Q. 20, 21, 37, 50
2   1, 31, 36, 54
3   11, 15, 17, 24, 32, 38
4   6, 9, 13, 18
5   4, 22, 23, 29, 30, 38, 58
6   1, 2, 3, 4, 26, 37, 39
7   10, 11, 12, 13, 28
8   1, 2, 3, 4, 58
9   2, 3, 4, 5, 6, 30, 56
10   1, 2, 3, 4, 8, 26

Applied anatomy
Examination
1   Q. 27
2   42
3   59
4   21
5   34
6   56
7   34
8   59
9   6
10   14

Paediatrics
Examination
1   Q. 7, 12, 16, 28, 30, 46
2   8, 48, 49
3   3, 48, 50
4   23, 24, 25
5   1, 4, 14, 22, 28, 39, 40,
       41, 42
6   23, 25, 26, 27, 28, 30,
       57, 58, 59
7   12, 16, 40, 41, 42, 43,
       46, 54
8   1, 3, 28, 34, 38, 39, 40,
       41
9   2, 4, 17, 45, 48, 51, 57,
       58, 59
10   27, 28, 29, 30, 37, 49,
       57, 58, 60

Genetics
Examination
1   Q. 31
2   13, 41
3   5, 36
4   15, 54
5   39
6   51, 55
7   1, 27
8   17, 37, 43
9   41, 51
10   55

Ophthalmology
Examination
1   Q. 33, 48
2   4, 21
3   26, 34, 37
4   17, 32
5   34, 42
6   56
7   21, 58, 59
8   44
9   7, 42
10   56

Statistics
Examination
1   Q. 35
2   60
3   60
4   60
5   60
6   60
7   60
8   60
9   43
10   59

Psychiatry
Examination
1   Q. 38, 51, 58
2   5, 24, 34, 57
3   45, 46, 47, 57, 58
4   50, 51, 52
5   18, 35, 36, 45
6   29, 30, 31, 32
7   37, 38, 39
8   40, 41, 42
9   25, 52, 53, 54, 55
10   35, 36, 37, 38

Reticuloendothelial diseases and malignancy
Examination
1   Q. 23, 24, 25, 54, 60
2   20, 46, 49
3   13, 30, 41
4   7, 25, 47, 58
5   6, 37, 50, 54
6   48
7   17, 56
8   7, 14, 18, 19, 54, 56
9   27, 48, 49
10   31, 32

Industrial diseases
Examination
1   Q. 16, 55
2   16
3   41
4   53
6   8, 49, 52
7   52

Physiology
Examination
1   Q. 57
2   19
3   42
4   27, 48
5   26
6   9, 14, 45
7   25
8   58
9   35, 60
10   19

Tropical diseases
Examination

1	Q. 14, 30
2	38
3	14, 51, 56
4	18, 51
5	30, 52
7	47, 49, 50
8	46, 47
9	21, 47
10	13

Signs and symptoms
Examination

1	Q. 22, 29, 34, 59
2	1, 3, 7, 31, 33, 39, 54, 59
3	26, 30, 33, 43, 44, 56
4	2, 3, 4, 6, 7, 8, 12, 13, 34, 39
5	5, 17, 19, 23, 33, 37, 45, 51
6	1, 14, 15, 18, 38, 39, 46, 56
7	10, 13, 20, 36
8	1, 3, 4, 16, 30, 31, 32, 50, 52, 53
9	10, 13, 16, 18, 44, 56, 58
10	2, 4, 5, 16, 46, 47, 53

Musculoskeletal and joint diseases
Examination

2	Q. 6, 22, 37
3	6, 10, 20, 23, 28, 40, 48
4	8, 38, 39
5	12, 13, 27, 31
6	17, 18, 46, 47, 53
7	22, 50, 51
8	12, 13
9	10, 18, 46, 57
10	52, 53

Toxicology
Examination

1	Q. 16
2	16, 51
3	41
4	42, 53
6	22, 49, 52
9	59

Immunology and allergy
Examination

1	Q. 60
3	30
5	6, 56
6	48, 50, 59
7	30, 44, 45, 49
8	19, 38
9	1, 15, 32, 48
10	23, 25

Chapter 5
The Trend and Bias of the Examination Questions: Common Topics Appearing in the Examination

Causes of papilloedema:
  Raised intracranial pressure as with:
    intracerebral abscess
    intracerebral tumour
    intracerebral haemorrhage
  Central retinal venous thrombosis as may be produced by:
    diabetes mellitus
    hypertension
    hyperviscosity syndromes
    primary blood disorders
  Retrobulbar neuritis—rarely
  Hypocalcaemia
  Carbon dioxide narcosis
  Superior vena caval obstruction

Loss of the red reflex is produced by:
  Cataracts
  Retinal detachment
  Vitreous haemorrhage

A red eye is produced by:
Blepharitis
Conjunctivitis
Iridocyclitis
Acute glaucoma
Non-traumatic/traumatic corneal ulcers

Causes of choroiditis:
Syphilis
Sarcoidosis
Tuberculosis
Toxoplasmosis
Collagen disorders
Injury
Idiopathic causes

Exophthalmos is produced by:
Primary thyrotoxicosis
Cushing's syndrome
Uraemia
Malignant hypertension
Superior mediastinal obstruction
Retrobulbar tumours/aneurysms
Cavernous sinus thrombosis
Severe myopia
Familial causes
Congenital defects, e.g. craniostenosis

Causes of ptosis:
IIIrd nerve palsy—commonest causes are:
  diabetes mellitus
  syphilis
  posterior communicating artery aneurysm
Sympathetic paralysis (Horner's syndrome)
Myasthenia gravis
Myopathy
  facioscapulohumeral type
  ocular type
Dystrophia myotonica
Congenital causes
Hysterical causes
Tabes dorsalis and general paresis of the insane

Splinter haemorrhages in the nails are found in:
Subacute bacterial endocarditis
Vasculitis, e.g. systemic lupus erythematosus
Trichiniasis
Traumatic injury to fingers

Drugs producing the L E syndrome (lupus erythematosus syndrome):
Hydralazine
Procainamide
Isoniazid
Anticonvulsants—phenytoin, methoin, troxidone, primidone, ethosuximide
Penicillin
Aminosalicylic acid
Reserpine
Aldomet (Alphamethyldopa)
Sulphonamides
Oral contraceptives
Phenylbutazone
Thiouracil
Griseofulvin
Tetracycline

Marked sweating is present in:
   Thyrotoxicosis
   Pulmonary tuberculosis
   Brucellosis
   Rabies

Sacroiliitis is a feature of:
   Reiter's disease
   Ankylosing spondylitis
   Psoriasis
   Enteropathic causes:
      Crohn's disease (regional ileitis)
      ulcerative colitis
      Whipple's disease

Sjögren's syndrome is associated with:
   Rheumatoid arthritis
   Scleroderma
   Polyarteritis nodosa
   Systemic lupus erythematosus

Causes of Raynaud's syndrome include:
   Scleroderma
   Cervical ribs
   Syringomyelia
   Tabes dorsalis
   Ergot poisoning
   Systemic lupus erythematosus
   Occupational—use of pneumatic drills
   Paroxysmal cold haemoglobinuria
   Peripheral neuropathy

Macroglossia is caused by:
   Cretinism/myxoedema
   Acromegaly
   Amyloidosis
   Mongolism

Causes of bilateral parotid gland enlargement:
Mumps–tender
Sarcoidosis
Lymphoma
Leukaemia
Tuberculosis
Syphilis
Mikulicz's syndrome

Hyperkeratosis of the palms and soles is produced by:
Bare-footed walking
Secondary syphilis
Keratoderma blenorrhagias of Reiter's disease
Hypovitaminosis A
Chronic inorganic arsenic poisoning

A rash in the butterfly distribution is produced by:
Light hypersensitivity:
   albinism
   porphyria
   pellagra
   drug-induced barbiturates
     sulpha drugs
     phenothiazines
Systemic lupus erythematosus
Acne rosacea
Tuberous sclerosis–adenoma sebaceum
Scleroderma

Miliary mottling on the chest x-ray is caused by:
Miliary tuberculosis
Sarcoidosis
Pneumoconiosis
Bilateral bronchopneumonia
Allergic aspergillosis
Haemosiderosis:
   primary idiopathic
   secondary, e.g. to mitral stenosis
Lymphangitis carcinomatosa

Causes of superior vena caval obstruction include:
Thymoma
Retrosternal goitre
Dermoid
Carcinoma of the bronchus
Aortic aneurysm
Constrictive pericarditis
Large pericardial effusion
Enlarged lymph glands from any of it's causes

Cannon 'a' waves are found with:
Complete heart block
Nodal tachycardia
Ventricular tachycardia

A small volume pulse is present with:
Mitral stenosis
Aortic stenosis
Severe pulmonary stenosis
Pericardial effusion/constrictive pericarditis
Shock state

Pulmonary fibrosis is caused by:
Tuberculosis
Bronchiectasis
Sarcoidosis
Pneumoconiosis
Collagen disorders:
    rheumatoid arthritis
    systemic lupus erythematosus
    scleroderma
Hamman–Rich syndrome

Transudates are found in:
Congestive cardiac failure
Renal diseases, e.g. nephrotic syndrome
Myxoedema
Hypoproteinaemia from any cause
Meig's syndrome
Severe anaemia

Iritis is associated with:
  Sarcoidosis
  Ankylosing spondylitis
  Rheumatoid arthritis
  Toxoplasmosis
  Ulcerative colitis
  Tuberculosis
  Syphilis

Cataracts are found with:
  Ageing
  Diabetes mellitus
  Trauma
  Maternal rubella
  Rickets
  Dystrophia myotonica
  Hypoparathyroidism
  Still's disease
  Galactosaemia
  Wilson's disease
  Marfan's syndrome

Masculine distribution of hair in a female is found in:
  Cushing's syndrome
  Virilizing adrenal tumours
  Pseudo–hermaphroditism
  Stein–Leventhal syndrome

Nodular hepatomegaly is found with:
  Post-necrotic cirrhosis
  Metastases to the liver
  Schistosomiasis
  Syphilis:
    gummata
    hepar lobatum of congenital syphilis

Causes of respiratory alkalosis:
Hysterical hyperventilation
Hypoxia
Intracranial causes:
    raised intracranial pressure
    meningitis
    haemorrhage
Pulmonary embolism
Pneumothorax
Salicylate overdosage

Causes of respiratory acidosis:
Obstructive airways disease—acute/chronic
Large pleural effusions
Guillain–Barré syndrome
Myasthenia gravis
Respiratory centre depression:
    drugs, e.g. morphine
    Pickwickian syndrome

Causes of metabolic alkalosis:
Excessive ingestion of alkalis
Hypokalaemia
Persistent vomiting

Causes of metabolic acidosis:
Uraemia
Renal tubular acidosis
Ureterosigmoidostomy
Diabetic ketoacidosis
Salicylate overdosage
Lactic acidosis
Shoshin form of beriberi with thiamine deficiency

Causes of hypercalcaemia:
  Primary/tertiary hyperparathyroidism
  Vitamin D toxicity
  Sarcoidosis
  Malignancy:
    metastatic to bone
    non-metastatic endocrine manifestation
  Milk–alkali syndrome
  Multiple myeloma
  Hyperthyroidism
  Idiopathic hypercalcaemia of infancy

Causes of hypocalcaemia:
  Hypoparathyroidism
  Due to hypoalbuminaemia
  Malabsorption syndrome
  Chronic renal failure
  Acute pancreatitis
  Renal tubular acidosis
  Hypovitaminosis D

Hypercholesterolaemia is found with:
  Pregnancy
  Nephrotic syndrome
  Diabetes mellitus
  Obstructive jaundice
  Myxoedema
  Primary biliary cirrhosis

Causes of hypernatraemia:
  Primary hyperaldosteronism
  Some patients with hyperosmolar non-ketoacidotic diabetic coma
  Diabetes insipidus
  Gastroenteritis especially in infants
  Intravenous saline infusions

Causes of hyponatraemia:
Addison's disease
Inappropriate secretion of antidiuretic hormone (ADH)
Diuretic therapy
Severe diarrhoea
Small gut fistulae
Water overload,
   e.g. cardiac failure
   nephrotic syndrome

Renal papillary necrosis is caused by:
Analgesic nephropathy
Tuberculosis of the kidney
Sickle-cell anaemia
Diabetes mellitus
Macroglobulinaemias

Autosomal dominant inheritance is seen in the following diseases:
Achondroplasia
Gardner's syndrome
Hereditary spherocytosis
Huntington's chorea
Intestinal polyposis
Marfan's syndrome
Neurofibromatosis
Polycystic kidneys (adult form)
Osteogenesis imperfecta
Hepatic porphyria
Tuberous sclerosis
Von Willebrand's disease
Ehlers–Danlos syndrome

Autosomal recessive inheritance of disease is associated with:
Albinism
Cystic fibrosis of the pancreas (mucoviscidosis)
Endemic goitrous cretinism
Familial amaurotic idiocy
Galactosaemia
Gaucher's disease
Glycogen storage disease
Phenylketonuria
Sickle-cell anaemia
Thalassaemia
Wilson's disease
Xeroderma pigmentosa

X-linked inherited diseases include:
Vitamin D-resistant rickets
Colour blindness
Glucose-6-phosphate dehydrogenase deficiency
Haemophilia A & B
Lesch–Nyhan syndrome
Duchenne's pseudohypertrophic muscular dystrophy
Agammaglobulinaemia

Causes of hypokalaemia include:
Long-term diuretic therapy without potassium replacement
Renal tubular acidosis
de Fanconi syndrome
Primary hyperaldosteronism (Conn's syndrome)
Cushing's syndrome
Adrenocorticotrophic hormone secreting tumours
Steroid therapy
Prolonged diarrhoea and vomiting
Purgative addicts

Kyphoscoliosis may be associated with:
Marfan's syndrome
Neurofibromatosis
Poliomyelitis
Tuberculosis of the spine
Ehlers–Danlos syndrome
Paget's disease of bone
Idiopathic—seen in the majority

Ophthalmoplegia may be caused by:
Migraine
Diabetes mellitus
Cranial arteritis
Exophthalmic ophthalmoplegia related to thyrotoxicosis
Myasthenia gravis
Cavernous sinus thrombosis/aneurysm
Intracranial tumours
Raised intracranial pressure
Syphilis
Meningitis

Causes of a carpal tunnel syndrome:
Pregnancy
Myxoedema
Rheumatoid arthritis
Amyloidosis
Acromegaly
Scleroderma
Systemic lupus erythematosus
Prolonged occupational pressure on the wrist

Acute ascending motor paralysis with retained sphincter function and a variable sensory loss is produced by:
  Guillain–Barré syndrome
  Infectious mononucleosis
  Viral hepatitis
  Acute intermittent porphyria
  Diphtheria
  Polyarteritis nodosa
  Toxic–
    triorthocresylphosphate
    stilbamidine

Causes of monocytosis include:
  Tuberculosis
  Infective endocarditis
  Brucellosis
  Malaria
  Trypansomiasis
  Ricketssial infections
  Hodgkin's lymphoma

Causes of eosinophilia include:
  Allergy
  Pemphigus
  Parasitic infections
  Polyarteritis nodosa
  Hodgkin's lymphoma
  Addison's disease
  Leukaemia, e.g. chronic myelocytic
  Myelofibrosis

Causes of acute generalized pruritis:
  Obstructive jaundice
  Internal malignancies
  Diabetes mellitus
  Severe renal insufficiency
  Lymphomas—Hodgkin's lymphoma
  Mycosis fungoides
  Primary polycythaemia—especially following a hot bath

Polyuria and polydipsia is caused by:
  Diabetes mellitus
  Diabetes insipidus
  Chronic renal failure
  Hypercalcaemia
  Hypokalaemia
  Compulsive water drinking

Hyperpigmentation is found in:
  Nelson's syndrome
  Addison's disease
  Hyperthyroidism
  Biliary cirrhosis
  Sprue
  Some cases of Cushing's syndrome

Paradoxical splitting of the 2nd heart sound is caused by:
  Left bundle-branch block
  Idiopathic hypertrophic subaortic stenosis
  Valvular aortic stenosis
  Some cases of patent ductus arteriosus
  Hypertensive heart disease with left ventricular failure
  Ischaemic heart disease with left ventricular failure

A higher incidence of carcinoma of the bronchus is reported with:
  Manufacture of coal gas
  Asbestos industry
  Mining of radioactive ores
  Refining of nickel
  Manufacture of chromates
  Processing of arsenic

Manifestations of hypersensitivity present in sarcoidosis are:
  Erythema nodosum
  Uveitis
  Arthritis
  Arteritis
  Thyroiditis

Side-effects of sulphonamides include:
Nausea and vertigo
Serum sickness
Erythema multiforme
Haemolytic/aplastic anaemia
Arthralgias
Hepatitis
Lesions resembling polyarteritis nodosa
Jaundice with kernicterus in babies

Furosemide produces the following side-effects:
Hypokalaemia
Pancreatitis
Thrombocytopenia
Neutropenia
Paraesthesiae
Skin rashes

Macular conditions of the skin are found in:
Vitiligo
Leprosy
Tinea versicolor
Morphoea

Papular conditions are seen in:
Early eczema
Psoriasis
Lichen planus
Urticaria pigmentosa
Syphilis
Acne vulgaris
Rosacea
Scabies
Molluscum contagiosum
Warts

Vesicular conditions are seen with:
Eczema–dermatitis
Cheiropompholyx
Tinea pedis
Erythema multiforme
Virus infections–variola, varicella, herpes simplex and
   zoster
Dermatitis herpetiformis
Herpes gestationis

Bullous conditions are seen with:
Burns
Frostbite/sunburn
Halogen drugs
Insect bites
Staphylococcal pemphigus neonatorum
Syphilis
Erythema multiforme
Dermatitis herpetiformis
Pemphigus
Pemphigoid
Epidermolysis bullosa

Pustular conditions are seen with:
Folliculitis
Acne vulgaris
Rosacea
Pustular psoriasis
Halogen eruptions
Variola
Infected eczema
Fungal infections

Causes of biological false–positive Wassermann reaction (W.R.) are:
Acute bacterial infection
Subacute bacterial endocarditis
Malaria
Leprosy
Autoimmune diseases, e.g. systemic lupus erythematosus
Acute viral infection (including smallpox)
Vaccination
Malnutrition

Causes of inappropriate anti-diuretic hormone (ADH) secretion:

(a) Malignancy:
      carcinoma of the bronchus (oat-cell type)
      carcinoma of the pancreas
      Hodgkin's lymphoma
(b) Infections:
      pulmonary tuberculosis
      acute pneumonia
      meningitis
(c) Drugs:
      chlorpromazine (Largactil)
      carbamazepine (Tegretol)
(d) Post head injury
(e) Acute intermittent porphyria

Causes of high urinary vanillyl mandelic acid level include:

Phaeochromocytoma
Clonidine withdrawal
Monoamine oxidase inhibitors ingestion
Alpha-Methyldopa therapy
Dietary factors: bananas, vanilla, tea, coffee, ice cream, chocolates
Phenothiazines
Tetracyclines

Causes of the lag storage type of glucose tolerance test:

Post gastric surgery
Thyrotoxicosis
Severe liver disease
Diabetes mellitus (early)
Occasionally in normal subjects

Causes of raised CSF protein above 2g/litre:

Guillain–Barré syndrome
Carcinomatous neuropathy
Neurofibromata (especially acoustic neuroma)
Meningitis:
    tuberculous
    acute bacterial
    fungal

Causes of a raised creatinine phosphokinase (CPK):
Myocardial infarction
Muscle injury (even following intramuscular injections)
Muscular dystrophies
Myxoedema
Severe physical exertion (including a severe asthmatic attack)
Alcoholism

Skin signs of internal malignancy include:
Acanthosis nigricans
Dermatomyositis
Pemphigoid
Erythroderma (exfoliative dermatitis)
Erythema gyratum perstans
Hyperpigmentation
Tylosis palmaris
Generalized pruritis
Acquired icthyosis
Hyperkeratosis of the palms and soles

Hypoparathyroidism may have the following features:
Raised intracranial pressure
Papilloedema
Cataracts
Calcification of:
    basal ganglia (common)
    choroid plexus
    cerebellum (dentate nucleus)
Psychosis
Dry coarse skin and brittle nails
Alopecia (axillary and pubic) with premature greying

Erythema nodosum is found with:
Bacterial infections:
  streptococcal
  diptheria
  primary tuberculosis (allergic manifestation)
  leprosy
  chancroid
  meningococcaemia
Viral infections:
  cat scratch disease
  lymphogranuloma venereum
  herpes simplex
Fungal infections:
  coccidiomycosis
  histoplasmosis
  blastomycosis
Drugs:
  contraceptive pill
  iodides
  bromides
  tetracyclines
Systemic diseases:
  rheumatic fever
  ulcerative colitis
  regional ileitis (Crohn's disease)
  systemic lupus erythematosus

Causes of gynaecomastia include:
Cirrhosis of the liver
Klinefelter's syndrome
Cushing's syndrome
Chorioepithelioma of the testis
Lepromatous leprosy
Bronchial carcinoma
Thyrotoxicosis
Drugs:
    long-term digitalis therapy
    spironolactones
    phenothiazines
    isoniazid (INH)
    adrenocorticotropic hormone/cortisol therapy
    hormonal therapy, e.g. as in oestrogen therapy in carci-
      noma of the prostate gland

Surgery for carcinoma of the lung is contraindicated by:
Evidence of metastatic lymph node involvement
Superior vena caval obstruction
Recurrent laryngeal/phrenic nerve infiltration
Pleural involvement due to the carcinoma
Distant metastases
Multicentric pulmonary lesions
Serious cardiopulmonary functional defects

Pulmonary infiltrates are found in:
Sarcoidosis
Pneumoconiosis
Malignancy, Carcinoma/
  Lymphoma
Histoplasmosis
Alveolar proteinosis
Polyarteritis nodosa
Cryptogenic fibrosing
  alveolitis
Pulmonary tuberculosis
Collagen disorders, e.g.
  scleroderma
Cystic bronchiectasis
Rheumatoid arthritis
Mucoviscidosis
Recurrent pulmonary
  oedema
Drugs, e.g. Busulphan,
  Bleomycin
  Nitrofurantoin, etc.

Chondrocalcinosis is found with:
Wilson's disease
Haemochromatosis
Ochronosis
Hyperparathyroidism
Diabetes mellitus

Protein-bound iodine is increased in:
Hyperthyroidism
Patients taking preparations containing iodides—
    cough mixtures
    Enterovioform
    asthma preparations
    x-ray contrast media
Pregnancy
Patients taking the contraceptive pill
Some cases of autoimmune thyroiditis
Patients taking:
    perphenazine
    clofibrate

Protein-bound iodine is decreased in:
Hypothyroidism
Malnutrition
Nephrotic syndrome
Cushing's syndrome/patients on corticosteroid therapy
Acromegaly
Patients with congenital absence of thyroid-binding globulin
Drugs therapy:
    mercurial diuretics
    androgens and anabolic steroids
    diphenylhydantoin therapy

High uptake of radio-iodine is seen in:
Hyperthyroidism
Dyshormogenesis in the thyroid gland
Iodine deficiency
Autoimmune thyroiditis (some cases)

Decreased radio-iodine uptake is seen in:
Primary/secondary hypothyroidism
Tri-iodothyronine/Thyroxine administration
Patients with a large stable iodine pool as is seen in:
    increased ingestion of iodine
        administration of contrast media (intravenous pyelo-
        gram, myelography, bronchography)
    Carbonic anhydrase inhibitor administration

Megaloblastic anaemia has been caused by:

Methotrexate	6-Mercaptopurine	Cyclophospha-
Cytosine arabi-	5-Fluorouracil	mide
nocide		
Primethamine	Triamterene	Pentamidine
Trimethaprim		
Hydantoins	Primidone	Phenobarbital
Para-amino		Colchicine
salicylic acid		
Neomycin	Alcohol	Oral contracep-
		tives

Causes of Parkinson's syndrome:
Idiopathic—paralysis agitans
Postencephalitic
Manganese poisoning
Hypoxia
Carbon monoxide poisoning
Repeated head trauma, e.g. as in pugilists
Familial
Drug intoxications:
    reserpine
    phenothiazines
    iron intoxication

The following drugs are all monoamine oxidase inhib-itors:

Iproniazid (Marsilid)	Pheniprazine (Catron)
Isocarboxazid (Marplan)	Nialamide (Niamid)
Phenelzine (Nardil)	Tranylcypromine (Parnate)
Pargyline (Eutonyl)	

Monoamine oxidase inhibitors interact with other substances listed below:

(a) Tyramine containing compounds:

Cheese	Coffee
Chicken liver	Pickled herring
Beer	Canned figs
Yeast	Broad beans
Wine	

(b) Drugs:

Amphetamine	Barbiturates
Alcohol	Meperidine
Morphine	Anticholinergic agents
Antidepressants:	Hypoglycaemic agents
Imipramine	Sedatives
Amitriptyline	Methyldopa
Sympathomimetic	Tryptophan
amines	Pethidine
Dopamine	Ephedrine
Antihistamines	
Reserpine	

Causes of pruritis include:

Uraemia

Anaemia

Liver diseases—obstructive jaundice, biliary cirrhosis

Systemic neoplasms

Reticuloses

Diabetes mellitus

Hyper-/Hypothyroidism

Senile pruritis

Pruritis of pregnancy (in the last trimester)

Urticaria/Allergy

Localized pruritis occurs in:

  Anogenital lesions

  Pruritis vulvae as in:

    diabetes mellitus

    vaginal candidiasis

    vaginal trichomoniasis

A mnemonic for the approximate incubation periods of various infectious diseases:

	Disease	Incubation period
D	Diphtheria	
I	Influenza	
C	Cytomegalovirus	1–7 Days
E	Erysipelas	
S	Scarlet fever	
T	Tetanus	
P	Poliomyelitis	
M	Measles	
E	Enteric fever (Typhoid)	7–14 Days
W	Whooping cough	
S	Smallpox	
C	Chickenpox	
R	Rubella	
U		
M	Mumps	14–21 Days
P		
S		

DICES   TP(MEWS)   CR(UMPS)

A mnemonic for the approximate time of first appearance of a rash in:

VERY	Varicella	Day 1
SICK	Scarlet fever	Day 2
PEOPLE	Pox (Small)	Day 3
MUST	Measles	Day 4
TAKE	Typhus	Day 5
EASE	Enteric fever (Typhoid)	Day 6
READILY	Rubella	Day 1–7

Appendix

Part I of the MRCP examination is held three times a year. For further details contact:

Royal College of Physicians of London,
Examination Office,
11 St Andrew's Place,
Regents Park
LONDON NW1 4LE

Royal College of Physicians of Edinburgh,
9 Queen Street,
EDINBURGH EH2 1JQ

Royal College of Physicians and Surgeons of Glasgow,
242 St Vincent Street,
GLASGOW G2 5RJ